WHAT TO DO FOR
A PAIN IN THE NECK

*The Complete Program for
Neck Pain Relief*

Jerome Schofferman, M.D.

Illustrations by Terry Toyama

A FIRESIDE BOOK
Published by Simon & Schuster

NEW YORK   LONDON   TORONTO   SYDNEY   SINGAPORE

FIRESIDE
Rockefeller Center
1230 Avenue of the Americas
New York, NY 10020

FIRESIDE and colophon are registered trademarks
of Simon & Schuster, Inc.

Designed by Stratford Publishing Services

Manufactured in the United States of America

10   9   8   7   6   5   4   3   2   1

Library of Congress Cataloging-in-Publication Data

Schofferman, Jerome A.
    What to do for a pain in the neck : the complete program for neck pain
relief / Jerome Schofferman ; illustrations by Terry Toyama.
        p. cm.
    Includes index
        1. Neck pain.   2. Neck pain—Treatment.   3. Neck pain—Exercise
therapy.   I. Title.

    RC936 .S28 2001
    617.5'3—dc21   2001020713

ISBN 0-684-87394-X

Acknowledgments

Over the years that I have been working in the field of spine medicine, I have met many wonderful and caring doctors. I can honestly say that most struggle as I do to find the best ways to help their patients. The best doctors have shared their insights and experiences with others who are trying to help. I am indebted to these doctors, who have been my teachers.

I have been extremely fortunate to work at the SpineCare Medical Group and the San Francisco Spine Institute. Dr. Arthur White founded the group and introduced me to the world of the spine. My other partners, Drs. James Reynolds, Noel Goldthwaite, Paul Slosar, and Garrett Kine, have supported me in my clinical work and encouraged my research and writing. The administrative staff at SpineCare, especially Jodie Faier, have supported me greatly as well.

Candice Fuhrman, my friend before she was my agent, felt there was a need for this book and encouraged me over and over to get it done. Her assistant, Elsa Dixon, edited several chapters and helped me through the process of getting the proposal finished. Gretchen Henkel, an editor of the highest caliber, helped me rework each chapter until it was clear, understandable, and free of too much medical jargon.

I would also like to thank the people at Simon & Schuster for their efforts and encouragement. Senior editor Caroline Sutton, her assistant, Nicole Diamond, and production editor Edith Baltazar contributed greatly to make my ideas a reality.

My patients have shown me what works and what does not. Without them, I would never have been inspired to do this work.

But, most of all, I thank my wife, Sally, for her enthusiasm and her love. Together we have learned that the couple that is not in motion rusts.

Contents

8   Contents

WHAT TO DO FOR

A PAIN IN THE NECK

1
Introduction

Neck pain has become one of the most common problems in our society. In fact, neck pain is so prevalent that we have come to accept it as a normal part of a busy life. Neck pain can affect anyone—office workers, computer scientists, writers, athletes, and manual laborers. Because you are reading this book, either you or someone you know probably has neck pain and may be frustrated by the lack of good information available. But help is at hand. Although there are some gaps in our scientific understanding of neck pain, we have sufficient knowledge to make useful recommendations about diagnosis and treatment to help most people.

We do not know exactly how many people suffer from neck pain, but the number is in the tens of millions. One study estimated that in any year, at least one-third of adults has an episode of neck pain! Even worse, approximately 15 percent of those people have chronic or recurrent neck pain. The goal of this book is to help you understand the causes of neck pain, and to provide you with effective and safe techniques to relieve it. Another goal is to provide you with guidelines to determine when or if you need professional care. And if you need help, the facts in this book should enable you to communicate better with your doctor, chiropractor, or physical therapist in order to optimize your care, and to become an active participant in it.

Neck pain is usually due to mechanical problems with one or more parts of the neck. It is rare for neck pain to be due to a serious illness like cancer or infection, but that said, the consequences of chronic and severe neck pain can be very serious. Some people are unable to work and may lose their jobs. Others cannot enjoy a social life, travel, or sports. Others may become irritable or depressed and develop marital and family problems. The financial consequences can also be dire: large amounts of money are spent on health care and disability payments each year because of neck pain.

Fortunately, there is hope for neck pain sufferers. There are highly qualified physicians, chiropractors, and physical therapists who specialize in spine problems. However, much of the up-to-date knowledge needed to help patients has not yet filtered down to the general orthopedist, family practitioner, or neurologist. Therefore, it is the responsibility of the person with neck pain to be informed. Even more important, the information and techniques in this book will help most people with neck pain get better without professional care.

People with chronic neck pain may initially try massage therapists, chiropractors, or acupuncturists. If they don't get better, they will see physical therapists, physicians, and finally surgeons. Frequently the initial treatment works and their condition improves. However, too often, pain recurs and the patient seeks help elsewhere.

In my practice, I see this pattern all the time and have learned that there are no quick and easy solutions to neck pain. It takes work and time to get better, and the patient must be an active participant. Treatment must be both aggressive and active. Too often, patients have had only passive treatment.

They have been treated with massage and manual therapy, heat packs and cold packs, and vitamins and herbs, but they have not been given the skills, knowledge, and training to play an active role in getting better. Fortunately, most people will respond to good conservative care that is scientifically based and sensitive to the needs of each patient.

However, even with excellent care, a small number of people still do not get better. Then the patient will need more aggressive forms of treatment that require the expertise of a spine specialist. Some patients will need spinal injections; some may even need surgery. Because each person is different, we need individualized treatment options. It is best to start simple and get more complex if necessary.

I never tell people to learn to live with the pain. Instead, I teach people how to overcome the pain. In this book, I will offer active and safe treatments that usually lead to improvement, or even total relief. I will offer advice based on my own extensive experience, coupled with the best scientific information available. However, I do not have any secrets or miracles. My treatment plan requires hard work and a commitment of time and energy. No single treatment works for everyone, so I will provide several treatment options. I will start with the fundamentals of strength training and body mechanics. If done correctly and diligently, these methods will often be effective treatment for most people. If not, these basic elements will provide the background necessary for the more aggressive treatments that I will recommend, most of which require professional care.

The premise of this book is simple. A person with neck pain must understand the anatomy and function of the neck. It is also very useful to know how our bodies transmit pain messages from the neck or other site of injury to the brain. Knowledge is power—power over pain. When you know the cause of the pain, you can develop treatment strategies that are specific for you. Some will be simple, such as rearranging your desk, workstation, and computer height or using your chair properly. Other strategies will be more complex, and will require a daily exercise routine and perhaps a few changes in lifestyle.

Most patients with long-standing neck pain will have flare-ups, despite being faithful to their programs. There are ways to help alleviate these intermittent flares, which I call "neck first aid." I will discuss the posture of the neck rest position, use of over-the-counter medications, proper use of ice, and a series of pain neutralization exercises, all geared to relieving the pain of flares.

In the remainder of this introductory chapter, I will present an overview of the problem of neck pain. I will introduce the subjects that I will discuss in detail later in the book. I recommend that you initially read or scan the book from beginning to end, and then return to the specific chapters that seem most important for you. This is especially true for the reader who is not familiar with medical or anatomic words and terms.

Neck Pain in the General Population

Almost everybody has had pain or stiffness in the neck at one time or another. In fact, we tend to accept neck pain as a normal part of life, and usually it goes away in a day or two without treatment. To try and determine the prevalence of neck pain in the general population, a group of medical researchers sent questionnaires to 10,000 people and asked if they had troublesome neck pain in the previous year, and, if so, how long it lasted. They found that 34 percent of those who answered the questionnaires had troublesome neck pain in the past year, and 14 percent had pain that lasted for more than six months!

Another survey found that at any one time, 22 percent of people have neck pain that is bothersome and two-thirds of people have had significant neck pain at some time in their lives. These studies make it clear that neck pain is a major health problem.

The Causes of Neck Pain: What Hurts and Why

The neck serves two basic functions. It is a pipeline for blood, nerves, food, and air, and it is a pedestal to hold up and support the head. Most of the problems that cause neck pain are due to damage to the pedestal and involve injuries to discs or joints. In addition, neck muscles may tire out and fatigue because of poor posture or overuse, contributing to the pain, but rarely being the underlying problem. When a person keeps his or her head in one position all day, there are stresses placed on the discs, joints, and/or muscles, resulting in pain.

When to See a Doctor

Many people are reluctant to go to a medical doctor for neck pain, partly because it seems like such a trivial problem, and are more likely to go to a massage therapist or chiropractor. However, if the pain persists, is very severe, or does not respond to chiropractic care or over-the-counter medications, it is time to see a physician.

There are also situations when you should go to a physician directly, rather than seeing another kind of health care provider first. If the neck pain is mild or absent, but there is severe pain in one or both arms, there may be pressure on a nerve in the neck, usually due to a disc herniation. This requires the evaluation of a doctor. If one or both arms become weak and you drop things or have difficulty lifting light objects, it is time to see a physician. The same is true if the neck pain becomes so severe that you are not able to go to work or do even simple household tasks. If there is a loss of bowel or bladder control, you should go to an emergency room immediately. None of these symptoms necessarily means that there is an emergency or that surgery is necessary, but they do mean that medical evaluation is required.

In other instances, it is optional to see a physician, and I make specific recommendations in chapter 11. However, if you are not getting better after three to six weeks of alternative health care, it is time to see a doctor. The doctor may need to order tests such as X-rays or an MRI scan. In addition, the doctor may be able to offer short-term relief by prescribing anti-inflammatory medications or other medications for pain. If the condition still does not improve, it may be necessary to do spinal injections, which can be very effective.

It is rare to need surgery for neck problems, but occasionally surgery is the best answer. Only a spine specialist can help you make this decision.

NECK-RELATED HEADACHES

It is estimated that about 16 percent of people suffer from headaches that occur sufficiently often to interfere with their lives. There are many types of headaches, including migraine headache, tension headache, cluster headache, and headache due to neck problems. A headache that occurs as a result of a disorder of the neck is properly called cervicogenic headache, but I use the term "neck-related headache" in this book.

Neck-related headaches occur in about 2.5 percent of people and account for about 15 percent of headaches that occur more than five days a month. They are almost as common as migraines, a type of headache that is often misunderstood. All types of headaches can cause severe pain, not just migraines. A migraine is a specific type of headache, not just a severe or "sick" headache. I believe that some people who are diagnosed with "tension-type headaches" and some who are diagnosed with migraine headaches actually have neck-related headaches. It is important to distinguish neck-related headaches from migraines and "tension-type" headaches when possible, because the treatments are different. The headache problem is important and discussed in detail in chapter 6.

Neck Pain After a Car Accident (Whiplash)

A significant number of people who are in motor vehicle accidents develop pain in the neck, shoulders, head, or the base of the skull. This group of symptoms is often called whiplash. Fortunately, most patients with whiplash recover in a few weeks, or at most a few months. However, about 10 percent to 15 percent of people do not get better, and they develop chronic pain. Whiplash is not a trivial problem. When neck pain occurs after a car accident, up to 30 percent of people still have pain one year later and 18 percent still have pain after two years.

There are many symptoms that may occur with whiplash in addition to neck pain, and at times they are sufficiently unusual to seem crazy. Some of these associated symptoms include sleep problems, poor concentration and memory, blurry vision, ringing in the ears, fatigue, and weakness.

The treatment for whiplash syndromes depends on the stage and degree of the problem and which structures have been injured. Almost all patients suffer from some form of soft tissue injury, usually strain of the muscles or ligaments. These strains or sprains heal over weeks or months and most patients improve. If pain persists, then it is likely that other structures, such as discs or joints, were also injured. In addition, patients who are encouraged to continue normal activities rather than resting also appear to do better.

There are many misunderstandings about the causes and treatments of whiplash. Perhaps the most controversial aspects are the effects of litigation on the rate of recovery. Whiplash is discussed in detail in chapters 4 and 5.

TREATMENT OF CHRONIC NECK PAIN

One ideal goal of medical care is primary prevention—avoiding a problem before it starts. The public is well acquainted with the primary prevention of heart disease, and we are all familiar with the recommendations to eat less fat, avoid cigarettes, and keep blood pressure normal. Similarly, primary prevention for neck pain requires exercising regularly and using good posture. Once a person has neck pain, it is obvious that primary prevention is no longer an option. The goal then shifts to pain relief and prevention of recurrences—called secondary prevention.

Proper care for the neck is simple in theory, but complicated to carry out in reality. The most important things a person can do to stay well include developing and maintaining good neck posture during rest and activity, and developing and maintaining sufficient strength in the muscles of the neck and upper back. In medical language, we refer to body positioning and posture as body mechanics. Good body mechanics must be maintained when you sit at a desk or in a chair reading, and when you participate in sports or work.

Most of us have neck muscles that are too weak to maintain good posture or to use good body mechanics for more than a few minutes at a time. Using good body mechanics and getting strong will solve the problem of neck pain for most people. The trick is to know what to do and how to do it. That is the essence of this book.

BODY MECHANICS AND EXERCISE

I have already mentioned that the most important things you can do to treat neck pain are to use good body mechanics and to get strong. The challenge is to find an exercise program that fits your own particular needs and lifestyle and to modify your body mechanics in ways that still let you do what you need to do.

The basic concept of body mechanics is surprisingly simple. The proper posture is one in which your chest is up, your chin is parallel to the floor, and your head is balanced between your shoulders, neither too far forward nor too far back. You must "sit tall." I am not suggesting a military posture, but one that is balanced and comfortable. You should be in this position whether sitting at a desk or playing sports. Motion of your head on the neck should occur primarily at the "hinge" at the top of the neck near the back of the jaw. The goal is to maintain this position standing up, sitting down, bending forward, and during all activities of daily living. Posture and body mechanics are discussed in detail in chapter 9.

The basics of neck muscle strengthening are also simple. You need to perform exercises on a daily basis to strengthen the muscles in the front of the neck, the back of the neck, and between the shoulder blades. All of these exercises can be done at home or in a gym, and I discuss the details of an exercise program in chapter 8.

PAIN MEDICATIONS

Most people with chronic neck pain have taken pain medications. Advertisers promote products that relieve all types of aches and pains. Each advertiser claims to have the best product, which leaves the consumer with an overwhelming amount of conflicting information. Fortunately, there are scientific answers to help the consumer decide which medications work best for each situation and which are safest.

There are three types of over-the-counter medications that are useful for neck pain. There are drugs that contain aspirin as the main ingredient. Examples of aspirin-based pain medications are regular aspirin, aspirin that is coated to partially protect the stomach, Excedrin, and Bufferin. There are products that contain acetaminophen as the main pain reliever such as Tylenol. Lastly, there are anti-inflammatory medications that contain either ibuprofen or naproxen. Some products add other active ingredients such as caffeine.

There are also many medications that are available only by prescription. These drugs are usually more potent than the medications sold over-the-counter. There are stronger anti-inflammatories, including some that can be taken just once a day, and provide twenty-four hours of relief. There are, in addition, medications that work on the brain to relieve pain. Other adjunctive medications that work on the complex pain pathways can be used in special circumstances and are very effective. Medications are discussed in detail in chapter 10.

DIFFERENT TYPES OF CARE

There are many treatments available for the person with neck pain. I divide the treatments into two general categories: passive and active. Passive treatments are things that a health care provider does to the patient. Active treatments are things the person does for himself or herself. Examples of passive treatments are massage, chiropractic, physical therapy that is only heat or ultrasound, and acupuncture. Active treatments include exercises and body mechanics training.

Passive treatments feel good while they are being administered. Although they rarely, if ever, do harm, they rarely do anything to improve the long-term outcome. Active treatments, such as those advocated in this book, can give a person the necessary skills and strengths to feel better and stay better.

Many people in this country seek alternative care rather than more traditional medical help from a physician. They may prefer remedies that are "natural" and that have been used for hundreds or thousands of years. Some alternative therapies do work, but most have never been tested in a scientific manner. I discuss alternative and complementary therapies in chapter 14 and chiropractors in chapter 12.

NECK PAIN AND SPORTS

Physical activity is generally good for neck pain. However, some sports can cause neck pain or make it worse when body mechanics are poor. I teach patients that it is not what you do, it is how you do it, and emphasize that most people can return to most sports when they are strong enough and trained to use proper body mechanics.

There are some sports that are difficult to do with neck pain. Bicycling requires careful attention to positioning on the bike so that the head is not bent too far forward or backward. Squash and racquetball both require a lot of twisting at the neck and are hard to do well while protecting the neck. The serve and overhead shots of tennis also are difficult to do properly. However, a person with neck pain can do all of these sports after instruction and practice in proper techniques. Neck pain in relation to sports and other recreational activities such as gardening is discussed in chapter 15.

The Psychology of Pain

Every person who has a neck injury, and especially those with chronic pain, have some form of psychological response. Some people feel anxious and might wonder if they will ever feel normal again. They worry that they will not be able to work, have a good family life, and play sports. Other people with chronic pain get depressed. They may suffer from problems sleeping and feel tired all the time.

There are also psychological problems that can make pain worse, but it is rare for pain to be purely psychological. However, whether the pain causes psychological problems or makes psychological problems worse, when psychological problems are present, they need to be treated. Many patients feel that if the pain got better, their psychological problems would go away, too. However, this is not always the case. Once established, the psychological problem has a life of its own. For a person to get better and stay better, both the physical injury and the psychological problems must be treated. I have discussed psychological problems and chronic pain in chapter 16, and I have outlined a program for self-help in chapter 17.

2

The Causes of Neck Pain: Where Does the Pain Come From?

OVERVIEW OF THE SPINE

The spine is a long linkage of bones, discs, muscles, and ligaments that extends from the base of the skull to the tip of the tailbone. The spine serves many functions. It supports the head and torso, protects the nerves and spinal cord, and allows for smooth and rhythmic function of the entire body during activity. It is designed so elegantly and is so versatile that a weight lifter can lift hundreds of pounds, a basketball player can float through the air, and a ballet dancer can bend into almost unimaginable positions.

The spine has three regions—an uppermost portion in the neck called the cervical spine, a middle portion in the torso called the thoracic spine, and the lowest part above the tailbone called the lumbar spine (figure 1). The major support is from the vertebrae, which are made of bone. There are seven cervical vertebrae, twelve thoracic vertebrae, and five lumbar vertebrae. The front of the vertebra is called the body and the back of the vertebra forms an arch. The linked vertebral bodies provide the major support for the spine and the linked arches surround and protect the delicate spinal cord and spinal nerves (figure 2).

In between each two adjacent vertebral bodies is a disc. Each disc acts as a shock absorber, but also stabilizes the vertebral bodies above and below it. In addition, ligaments and muscles provide support.

PRACTICAL ANATOMY OF THE NECK

The neck is basically a tube, but it is not hollow. Inside the neck, there is the spinal column that supports the head. The bones and cartilage of the spinal column surround and protect the spinal cord and nerves. Muscles and ligaments surround the spinal column and function like guy wires to keep it from toppling over by the forces placed upon it. In addition to supporting the head, the neck serves as a passage or conduit for air, food, nerves, and blood vessels.

The neck is made of layers, with each layer encircling the one beneath it like the rings of an onion. The skin is the outermost layer and the spinal cord is innermost. Pain might arise from any layer, and so I will discuss each layer and the types of injuries that might affect each one. Because many of the structures of the neck have rich nerve supplies, injury or damage to almost any one can cause pain. However, in most instances, chronic neck pain is due to mechanical breakdown of the discs or facet joints, with damaged ligaments or muscles making much less of a contribution.

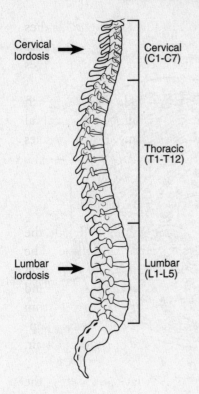

Cervical lordosis →

Cervical (C1-C7)

Thoracic (T1-T12)

Lumbar lordosis →

Lumbar (L1-L5)

Figure 1
The spinal column is divided into cervical (neck), thoracic (upper back), and lumbar (lower back) regions. The lowest curve (lumbar lordosis) forms the foundation for the rest of the spine.

Figure 2
Cross-sectional view of the cervical spine as if you were lying facedown. It shows the relationships between a disc with its anulus, nucleus, and small nerves; the spinal cord, and spinal nerve roots.

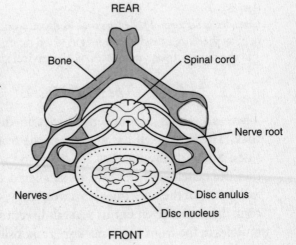

REAR

Bone

Spinal cord

Nerve root

Nerves

Disc anulus

Disc nucleus

FRONT

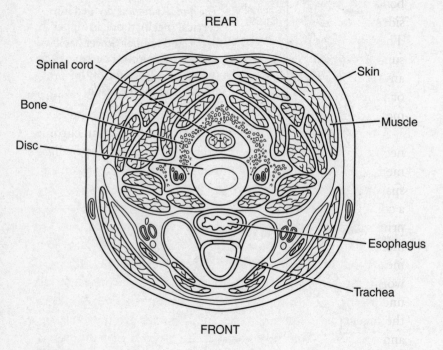

REAR

Spinal cord

Skin

Bone

Muscle

Disc

Esophagus

Trachea

FRONT

Figure 3

Cross-sectional view of the entire neck as if you were lying facedown. It depicts the skin, muscles, esophagus (food pipe), trachea (airway); and the bones, discs, and nerves of the cervical spine.

The Neck Muscles

There are about two dozen muscles in the neck and upper back. The neck itself has muscles in the front, back, and both sides. Some of the muscles are large and near the surface so they can be felt easily. Others are smaller, deeper, and harder to feel. Some of the neck muscles have a single function, but most contribute to movement in several directions. In general, the muscles in the front of the neck are responsible for bending the head forward (flexion), the muscles in the rear of the neck for bending the head backward (extension), and the muscles on the sides of the neck for bending to the left or right, and rotating. The muscles between the shoulder blades form a platform that supports the neck and head. Damage, strain, or other injury to any of the muscles of the neck can cause pain. Weakness in one or more muscle groups forces the discs and joints to support more weight, which may lead to damage of these structures.

Most people, including most doctors, think that chronic neck pain usually is due to problems in the muscles or ligaments, and that increased muscle tension causes pain and spasm. This view is only partially correct and overly simplifies a complex problem. There are two categories of muscle pain— primary and secondary. Primary muscle pain means that the muscles are the major cause of the pain. Secondary muscle pain means that muscles are painful and in spasm because they are working too hard to support the head and to protect injured underlying structures. The muscles are not the weak links in the chain; the joints and discs are. Muscles are more elastic, and are better able to withstand the stresses of daily living, than the joints or discs. In order to determine if muscle pain is present, and whether it is primary or secondary, one must evaluate the pain with respect to its intensity, its mechanism of onset, and those factors that aggravate or alleviate the pain.

Primary muscle pain is usually mild or moderate, but it is rarely severe. Based on my clinical experience and a thorough review of the available scientific evidence, I believe that most instances of moderately severe to severe chronic neck pain are due to damage to structures that lie deeper in the neck. The muscles may contribute to the pain, but only as a secondary problem.

In some instances, primary muscle pain may begin suddenly, such as after a car accident. Although the pain can occur immediately, most often it begins after several hours, and occa-sionally only after a few days have passed Muscle pain after an acute injury subsides rather quickly, usually in a few weeks. Certainly, it does not last for more than three to four months, unless there is something else wrong that sustains the muscle pain, such as an underlying joint or disc injury, or poor posture and work habits.

In other instances, primary muscle pain has a more gradual onset, most commonly in people whose work requires sus-tained, poor postures. Examples include working at a com-puter all day or holding a telephone between the ear and the shoulder for long periods of time. These ergonomic problems usually are mild in the beginning of the workday, and worsen as the day goes on. They get better on vacations and weekends. They are annoying, but not severe.

The function of the neck muscles is to maintain good pos-ture by holding the head up and erect. In turn, good neck pos-ture protects the joints and discs and keeps the neck muscles from overworking. When muscles are sustained in these pro-longed states of contraction, they tire, build up waste products, and hurt. If the muscles are weak, they fatigue more quickly and pain occurs sooner, no different from any other over-worked muscle that is not strong enough to do its job. If there is an underlying injury to deeper structures of the neck, the muscles must work even harder to protect these injured parts, and they fatigue more quickly. Then there is pain from the muscles in addition to the pain from the deeper injured struc-tures.

One of the basic treatments of neck pain is to strengthen the neck muscles in order to be able to develop and maintain excel-lent posture and body mechanics. When these goals are met, pain is often relieved. It may seem confusing to state that although muscles are not the primary cause of neck pain, strengthening the muscles will help relieve the pain, but it works. Strong muscles are necessary for good posture, and good posture is necessary for underlying structures to heal.

The Motion Segment

The basic functional unit of the spine is called the motion segment (figure 4). The entire spine is made up of a vertical stack of these segments. Each motion segment is composed of two adjacent vertebral bodies made of bone, one on top of the other, but separated by a disc. A disc has two parts. The center of the disc is the nucleus (nucleus pulposus) and is made of protein and water. The outer part of the disc is the anulus fibrosus, which is cartilage, and tough like gristle. Each motion segment

Figure 4

A motion segment consisting of two vertebrae and the one disc and two facet joints between them, side view. Also pictured are the spinal cord and a spinal nerve root.

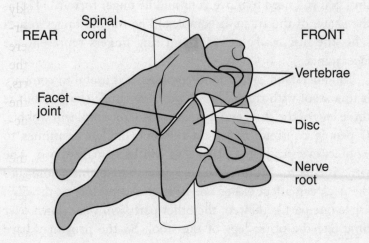

has two joints in the rear, one on each side, called facet joints (or more properly called zygapophyseal joints), and has ligaments and muscles. There are seven vertebrae and six discs in the neck. There is no disc between the first and second vertebrae.

A motion segment is numbered by its two vertebrae, starting from the top and moving down. For example, the motion segment that contains the fourth and fifth cervical vertebral bodies is called C4/5. The next segment down would be called C5/6. The fifth cervical vertebra is a part of both C4/5 and C5/6 motion segments. The disc and facet joints are named in the same manner. The disc that lies between the fourth and fifth vertebral bodies is called the C4/5 disc, and the two facet joints at the same level would be termed the left or right C4/5 facet joints respectively.

The disc and the facet joints make up a "tri-joint complex." In order to visualize this, place your arm parallel to the floor and bend your wrist down to a 30- to 45-degree angle. Place the tips of your index, middle, and ring fingers on the surface of a table so that only the tips of all three fingers touch it. To do this, you will need to move your middle finger forward. This is the shape of the tri-joint complex. The middle finger represents the disc, and the index and ring fingers represent the facet joints.

To understand the tri-joint complex, it is useful to compare it to a stool with three legs. If there is damage to one of the three legs of the stool and it is shortened, the stool will wobble. If people continue to sit on the stool and it continues to wobble, eventually the other legs will be damaged, too. The same is true for progressive neck pain. The primary injury to the neck can affect either one or both facet joints or the disc. Once one part is injured, the other parts will wear down over time like the other legs of the stool. So the pain may have begun with one part of the motion segment, but over other parts will also hurt.

Facet Joints (Zygapophyseal Joints or Z Joints)

The facet joints can be a troublesome cause of neck pain. In chronic whiplash, the facet joints are the single most common cause of neck pain. The facet joints are designed to allow smooth motion for bending forward, bending backward, and rotating. The joints also limit excess motion. The facet joints can be injured easily. In some people, when the joints begin to wear, they make popping or cracking noises when the head is turned; noises that are not dangerous can be compared to cracking knuckles.

It is instructive to extend the knuckle analogy to the facet joints to explain how they can cause pain. If you forcefully bend a finger knuckle backward beyond its normal range, it will hurt. When you release it, the pain usually subsides, but after a few hours, inflammation begins and pain recurs. Then, even normal range of motion of the knuckle is painful. Similarly, if you gently bend your knuckle backward just beyond its normal range, it may not be painful immediately, but if you hold it there long enough, it will become inflamed and begin to hurt. Then, once again, even normal range of motion will hurt. These are examples of what often happens to the facet joints. The forceful knuckle bend is like a whiplash. The gentle knuckle bend is like sitting for long periods with bad posture in which the facet joint sustains a position that is just beyond its limit.

The facet joints have a rich nerve supply. The nerve that conducts signals from the joint to the spinal cord is called the medial branch of the dorsal ramus of the spinal nerve, or "medial branch" for short. When we test to see if a facet joint is a cause of pain, we numb this specific nerve (see chapter 3). If the pain goes away when the joint is numb, that joint is most likely the source of the pain. If the pain does not go away, that joint is not the cause of the pain.

Facet joints can wear painfully or painlessly. There is a very poor correlation between the appearance of the joint on X-ray, MRI scan, or CAT scan, and whether it hurts. A joint can look terrible on an X-ray or scan and be painless, or it can look normal and be a source of pain. The only test to see if the joint is a cause of pain is the medial branch block discussed above.

Discs

Most people have heard of a herniated disc or slipped disc, but there is much more to the disc story. The disc is a simple structure, but it can wreak havoc. Each disc has an inner core called the nucleus pulposus (often referred to simply as the nucleus), and an outer shell called the anulus fibrosus (also called the anulus). As already discussed, each disc lies between two vertebral bodies, one above and one below. The disc functions as a joint, one part of the tri-joint complex. It allows movement and flexibility of the vertebrae above and below, and at the same time provides a great deal of stability against excess motion. Discs also provide shock absorption.

The anulus is made up of collagen, a strong and tough substance. The anulus surrounds the nucleus and keeps it in its proper place, and also plays a major role in stabilizing the motion segment. The anulus is much thicker in the front of the disc and very thin in the rear, where most injuries occur. In the normal disc, the outer one-third of the anulus has nerve endings that are sensitive to pressure and possibly inflammatory chemicals. In the low back, it has been shown that with discs that have been damaged for a long time, the nerve endings proliferate and grow inward toward the nucleus. Although this has not been evaluated in the neck, it is presumed that the same type of reaction may occur.

The anulus can be torn or cracked either by an acute injury, or by chronic strain. Anulus tears and cracks may cause inflammation as well as a decrease in the structural integrity of the disc that is so necessary to provide full support. The weakened anulus renders the disc susceptible to more compression than a normal disc under similar loads. In turn, the increased compression causes more stimulation of the nerve endings in the anulus and can result in pain under circumstances in which a normal disc would not hurt.

Fortunately, anulus tears usually heal without residual effects. However, recurrent tears may lead to loss of some of the water from the nucleus, which is part of the degenerative process. In most individuals, discs degenerate painlessly, as a normal part of the aging process. However, in others, discs hurt when they degenerate, and become a cause of chronic neck pain. The pain comes from the stimulation of the nerve endings in the anulus, not because the disc pushes on any big nerves. This is one of the most poorly understood facts about neck pain.

The classic disc problem is a herniated disc, which means the nucleus has moved backward through cracks and tears in the anulus and now is sticking out (figure 5). The anulus may be completely torn, or just thinned out enough to let the nucleus distend it. A disc herniation can cause pain by pushing on a nerve or on the spinal cord.

Another way a damaged nucleus can lead to pain is biochemical. The damaged nucleus makes inflammatory chemicals, which spread to the nerve fibers in the anulus and render them even more sensitive. It then takes less pressure on the anulus to cause pain.

When the nucleus is pushing on a large nerve root, it can cause arm pain. This occurs when the herniation is off to one

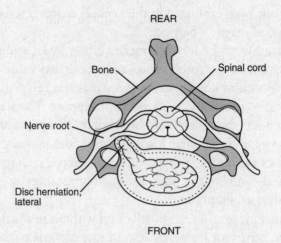

Figures 5 and 6

Disc herniations. Figure 5: A disc herniation off to one side (lateral), which pushes against a nerve root. Lateral disc herniations may cause both arm and neck pain. Figure 6: A disc herniation in the midline (central) does not push on a nerve root. Midline disc herniations may cause neck pain, but rarely cause arm pain.

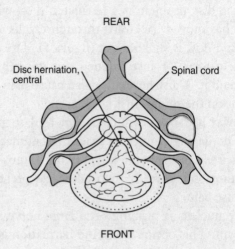

side or the other. The location of the pain would depend on which nerve is being pushed. If the nucleus herniates straight back, it usually causes much more neck pain than arm pain (figure 6).

Nerve Root Entrapment

All physicians agree that pressure on a nerve root can cause pain. The normal nerve root carries messages from the hand or arm to the brain, and then back again. It is through the nerve root that we have the sense of touch in our hands, and that we can make our muscles move. However, if a nerve is being compressed or squeezed, various things can happen. If the pressure is mild or moderate, there may be pain, numbness, or tingling. If the nerve is more severely compressed, there may be weakness of the muscles served by that nerve. On rare occasions, there can be weakness with little or no pain.

A nerve can be compressed in several ways, including a disc herniation, or bone spurs. When a disc degenerates over years, bone spurs form. If the bone spurs grow in the front of the disc where there are no nerves, it just makes for an ugly X-ray. However, if the bone spurs grow into the nerve canal, the nerve can be compressed and cause pain, weakness, and/or reflex loss.

Spinal Cord Compression

The spinal cord is the conduit for electrical messages to travel from the nerves of different parts of the body up to the brain, and then down again from the brain via the nerves to the body parts. Spinal cord injury interrupts the flow of nerve messages. There are various degrees of spinal cord injury. Some cause only minor symptoms, but others are severe and can cause paralysis.

Most often, the type of spinal cord compression that we see in the office setting has taken place over many years. As discs and joints of the motion segment wear out, bone spurs develop. Gradually, these bone spurs can intrude into the central spinal canal, and begin to compress the spinal cord. In addition, on rare occasions, we see a large disc herniation that compresses the spinal cord.

SYSTEMIC ILLNESSES THAT AFFECT THE NECK

Skin

We usually do not think of the skin when we think of the causes of neck pain, but some skin conditions are painful. Most often, when pain is due to a skin condition, it is obvious because there is a rash or lesion. Common examples of painful skin problems include shingles, bad sunburn, or infection.

One skin condition that can cause severe neck pain is shingles. Shingles is due to a viral infection from herpes simplex, the virus that causes chicken pox. Usually, the virus is acquired during childhood, lies dormant for many years, and then is activated by stress, another systemic illness, or a weakened immune system, and spreads to the skin through the nerves. The skin becomes very painful, and extremely tender to even the lightest touch. Even the touch of a bedsheet can cause severe pain. In most instances, the infection clears, either spontaneously or with medications, and the pain abates. However, in some people, the rash clears but severe pain remains, a condition called postherpetic neuralgia.

If you suspect shingles, it is important to see a doctor promptly, because early treatment with antiviral drugs may prevent postherpetic neuralgia. Once established, postherpetic neuralgia may be difficult to treat.

Thyroid Gland

In addition to its role as a supporting structure, the neck contains the thyroid, which is located in the front of the neck, just under the skin and superficial muscles. Most thyroid disorders do not hurt. However, if there is an infection in the gland (called thyroiditis) or an inflammatory metabolic disturbance, there can be pain. When the thyroid gland is the cause of pain, the person usually feels ill with fever, weight loss, diarrhea, or palpitations. If these symptoms are present with neck pain, it is important to see a physician.

Throat

Almost everyone has had a sore throat. With a bad streptococcal infection ("strep throat") or viral infection, there will be obvious pain in the throat. However, if the lymph glands get inflamed, there can also be pain throughout the front and back of the neck and possibly behind the jaws. Again, this problem is usually obvious.

Heart

On rare occasions, pain that arises from the heart can be felt in the neck, usually in the jaw area. It has a sudden onset, usually during or after vigorous activity. Often, it occurs in middle-aged and older individuals who usually have risk factors for heart disease, such as cigarette smoking, high blood pressure, high cholesterol, or strong family history.

Pain Physiology

The nervous system is truly remarkable. We each have a highly developed system that thinks, governs all of our bodily functions, senses our environment, and moves our muscles. Our bodies have evolved a system of sense organs that are specific for touch, taste, sight, sound, and smell. Stimuli from the environment as well as from our internal organs travel along a complex pathway that uses electricity and biochemicals to relay the messages up to the brain. Then the brain interprets the signals, modifies them, and sends back a response. All of this happens in less than the blink of an eye.

We also have developed a pain system. In the evolution of the human, pain was a warning signal that something was wrong. It told the animal (even the human animal) that there was an injury, and served to remind the animal to get out of harm's way. The pain system is not a simple highway of messages, but is in many ways more complex. As we developed the abilities to think, feel, and interpret, the pain system evolved as well. The stimulus that we interpret as pain gets modified all along this inner information highway on the way to the brain. The way this occurs is the subject of pain physiology.

Definition of Pain

Because each of us has experienced it, it might seem simple to define pain, but it is not. Scholars have been arguing over a definition of pain for years, and the International Association for the Study of Pain formed a committee that eventually agreed on a definition of pain. They defined pain as: "an *unpleasant sensory* and *emotional* experience associated with *actual or potential tissue damage* or described in terms of tissue damage" (italics mine).

Several things are apparent from this definition. Pain is, by definition, always unpleasant. There is a sensory component, meaning that there has been stimulation of the nervous system. There must be some type of emotional response to that stimulation, such as fear, anxiety, or depression. Finally, there is, or was, damage to some part of the body, or at least the stimulation was strong enough that it might cause damage.

Obviously, you do not need a definition of pain to know when you hurt. However, the cause of pain is often a mystery. Pain is not one of the five senses, and it does not behave like vision, hearing, smell, touch, or taste. Pain is more of an experience than a sense. The original stimulation is modified by psychological, social, and environmental factors.

Pain Neurology

In order for us to experience pain, there must be damage (or the immediate potential for damage) to some part of the body. This damage stimulates the nerves in that part of the body, which begins the transmission of the message. Then the resulting electrical signal must be transmitted from the site of damage to the brain. Along the route to the brain, the signals move along nerves until they reach the major conduction trunk, the spinal cord. The signals then are conducted up the spinal cord to the brain. At many points along the way, other nerves enter the spinal cord. At each entry point, the original pain signal can be modified. In some instances, the signal is turned down, resulting in less pain. In other instances, it is turned up, resulting in pain that is worse.

Let us consider a few examples. When an animal suffers a cut, it may lick the wound. The licking, among other things, provides another stimulus to the nervous system over other nerves, and modifies the original signal, which may decrease the pain. Other examples include rubbing your elbow or knee when it has been banged or bumped. Rubbing the injured part sends in another signal to the nervous system that modifies the original injury. Tiger Balm and other salves that stimulate the skin send messages to the brain via the spinal cord, and may decrease the pain signal and pain intensity.

Other inputs can modify the stimulus, many of which affect the brain, the final endpoint for the pain message. Many inputs from the body arrive at the brain simultaneously. In addition, the brain is the seat of our emotions, and our emotional state is a major influence on the processing and interpreting of these messages. If a person is depressed when the pain signal arrives, the pain may seem worse. If a person is in a good mood, the pain may seem less severe. If you do not get a good night's sleep, pain may be worse the next day. If you are able to distract yourself with a good book, movie, or conversation, the pain seems less.

Finally, the brain sends a pain message back down the conduit to the injured part. Pain is then perceived in the area of the body that was injured, but it is really experienced in the brain.

Pain Tolerance and Threshold

It is clear that the same injury causes severe pain in some people, and minimal or no pain in others. There are complex explanations for this phenomenon. Some of the issues have already been addressed—pain signals can be decreased or increased all along the transmission pathways, and the interpretation of the signals is somewhat dependent on our emotional state.

However, interestingly, all of us sense pain at about the same stimulation intensity. In a laboratory, heat can be applied to skin in carefully regulated degrees. Almost everyone feels pain at about the same temperature. The stimulation intensity at which most of us agree is painful is called the pain threshold.

However, each person is somewhat different with respect to the intensity and duration of the stimulation that we can tolerate. This is called pain tolerance. All of the factors that we have discussed, particularly the psychological ones, influence our pain tolerance. Pain threshold is relatively fixed.

Referred Pain

It is common for a person to feel pain in an area of the body distant from the part that has been injured, a phenomenon that occurs for several reasons. One, as previously discussed, is that there is compression or pressure on a nerve root, and this is the nerve that conducts signals to and messages from that area. The other phenomenon is called referred pain—pain that occurs in a location downstream from the injury.

Referred pain is actually quite common. Perhaps the best-known example is the pain from a heart attack. A person who is experiencing a heart attack usually will feel chest pain. However, it is common to also feel pain in an arm, usually the left one. Obviously, there is nothing wrong with that arm. It is that the nerves that come from the arm and the nerves that come from the heart enter the spinal cord at about the same location, and then travel together up to the brain. Since the signals have intermingled, the brain does not quite know where the message first arose and sends a pain message back down to both the chest and the arm.

When considering neck problems, there are two common locations for referred pain—the arm and between the shoulder blades. Referred arm pain does not necessarily follow the pattern of the nerve exactly, and so might be confusing. There may even be tingling and a feeling of deep numbness, confusing things even more. Pain between the shoulder blades is very common when there are neck problems. Often, patients have been erroneously told there is a rib out of alignment in the area of pain, because sites of referred pain can be tender. Interestingly, when the neck pain improves, pain in the arm and between the shoulder blades gets better as well.

3

How to Make the Diagnosis of Neck Pain

Almost any structure in the neck can cause pain when it is injured (see chapter 2). Interestingly, except for rare emergencies, it is seldom necessary to know the exact cause of pain to begin treatment, because most patients will improve no matter what the cause of the pain. However, when a patient is not getting better, finding the cause of the pain is necessary in order to plan more aggressive treatment. An accurate diagnosis is formed based on the medical history, physical examination, and specialized tests.

The Medical History

In medicine, "the history" is also called the history of the present illness, and refers to the information obtained from a patient. The purpose of taking a history is to help the physician make a working diagnosis, determine if testing is needed, and plan treatment. A complete medical history includes the details of the current problem, as well as a brief description of general health status, family illnesses, psychological issues, past injuries, past medical or surgical illnesses, and cigarette or alcohol use. For neck pain, the history amounts to "the story of the pain" and includes how the pain began; the mechanism of injury, if any; prior episodes of similar pain; things that make pain better or worse; and the effects of head and neck motion.

There are many ways to take a history. Some doctors like to start with the onset of the pain and work forward to the current status. Others start with a description of the current pain and then review the mechanism of injury or onset of pain. Some physicians prefer an "open-ended history," in which the patient describes the problem. Others use a "directed history," in which the doctor asks specific questions. Many spine specialists use questionnaires designed to ask about the most important aspects of neck pain.

Onset of Pain

The way the pain began may provide clues to the diagnosis. Some people know exactly when their neck pain began because a specific accident or injury caused it. Traumas such as a motor vehicle accident, a fall, a bicycle accident, or a blow to the head may injure discs or facet joints, and may cause muscle spasm.

Neck pain that occurs as a result of a car accident is commonly called whiplash (see chapter 4). Most often, the neck pain begins hours or days after an accident. Eighty percent of the time, the pain improves in several weeks. However, it may last as long as four to six months, and most research studies show that about 10 percent to 20 percent of people are left with some degree of chronic neck pain.

Some people with neck pain after an accident recover initially, but develop pain again five to ten years later. In these cases, the accident may have caused a minor injury to a disc that appeared to have healed. However, the injury may have caused the injured disc to degenerate much faster than normal and it eventually causes pain many years later.

Neck pain can develop after being struck on the head by a falling object or hitting the head on an overhang when getting up from bending over. The impact sends forces down the neck and injures discs or joints. Many people with these types of injuries may also suffer subtle damage to the brain (called traumatic brain injury) and develop changes in their mood, memory, or thought processes.

When the onset of pain is more gradual, the cause may not be as clear. Your usual work and recreational activities, especially those that make pain worse, can provide your doctor with clues to the cause of the pain. For instance, pain may be due to cumulative trauma from frequent repetitions of the same activity or from working in one position all day long. Working at a computer, laying carpet, painting walls and ceilings, or gardening are examples of repetitive activities that can cause trauma over time.

Description of the Pain

A description of pain includes its severity, location, frequency, and duration. Severe neck pain usually is due to a disc tear (also called an anulus tear) or herniation, possibly with pressure on a nerve root. Strong pain medications may be needed temporarily to provide relief while evaluation and other treatments are in progress. Mild or moderate pain is not very specific—that is, it can be difficult to diagnose its source without specialized tests. Severe arm pain suggests a disc herniation.

The location of neck pain may not always help lead to a specific diagnosis. The location of arm pain, however, can be more helpful because when a nerve is being compressed, the arm pain follows the path of that nerve. Pain that radiates down one arm and follows the path of a specific nerve suggests a disc herniation that is putting pressure on a nerve. Pain one-half to one inch to either side of the middle of the back of the neck is often attributed to muscle pain, but this may not be the whole story. The facet joints lie directly under the muscles, and when the muscles are pressed, they are compressed against the facet joints. Tenderness may be coming from joints, muscles, or both. It is common for pain from discs or facet joints to be referred, or felt at a different site, such as the shoulder blades, the upper arm, the base of the skull, or the head.

Most neck problems due to injured discs, joints, muscles, or other soft tissues cause pain in the back of the neck. When pain is in the front of the neck, it may be due to a medical problem such as an infection in the lymph node, thyroid gland, or salivary gland. Persistent pain in the front of the neck, especially if associated with fever, difficulty swallowing, or weight loss, may require consultation with an internist.

Constant pain usually causes greater disruption than intermittent pain. If you have pain that comes and goes, carefully consider your usual activities of daily life with special attention to those things that make pain better or worse. This information may lead to a correct diagnosis and better treatment.

Mild to moderate pain of recent onset usually is treated with exercises, modification of activity, and anti-inflammatory medications. However, pain that has been present for more than three or four months may require a detailed evaluation, because it is unlikely to improve without specific diagnosis and treatment.

Most pain changes in intensity or location depending on the position of the head and neck. If your pain is worse after prolonged periods of reading, writing, or computer work, you may have a disc problem. Pain that is made worse by looking overhead may be originating from an inflamed facet joint.

Patterns of Pain

In chapter 2, I discussed most of the many potential causes of neck pain. In addition to discs, bones, muscles, and other soft tissues, there are nerves that carry the pain signals from the neck, down the arm to the hands and fingers. There is a complex interweaving and bundling of nerves and nerve signals, which sometimes makes it difficult to determine the cause of the pain by its pattern and distribution. However, there are some patterns that are consistent from patient to patient.

RADICULAR PAIN PATTERN

Arm pain associated with decreased muscle strength or a loss of reflex or sensation, and that follows the distribution of a single nerve, is called radiculopathy. The distribution of a single nerve from the neck is called a dermatome (figures 7 and 8). One cause of arm pain is compression of a nerve root in the neck by a disc herniation or by bone spurs that have narrowed the nerve root canal. When this occurs, the pain in the arm will follow a single dermatome. However, it is more common for arm pain to be due to referred pain, which is "cross talk" between nerves in the spinal cord, and discussed in chapter 2.

The distribution and location of arm pain may suggest which segment of the neck has been injured. As described in chapter 2, the neck has seven discs, each of which lies between one vertebra above it and another below it. Discs are named according to these two adjacent vertebrae, so the disc that lies between the fourth (C4) and fifth (C5) vertebrae is called C4/5. Nerve roots exit between two cervical vertebrae and are named for the lower one, so, for instance, the nerve that exits at the C4/5 disc level is called C5. The distributions of the C5, C6, C7, and C8 nerves generally are consistent from person to person, and are also the nerves that are injured most often. The distribution of these nerves is shown in figures 7 and 8.

The C5 nerve originates between the C4 and C5 vertebrae, travels to the outside of the upper arm to the region of the deltoid muscle, and may also spread to the biceps muscle. When C5 is compressed or irritated, there may be pain or numbness in the deltoid muscle on the outside of the upper arm, continuing down the thumb side of the forearm. If there is significant C5 nerve root injury, there may be weakness when raising your arm sideways, away from your body.

The C6 nerve originates from between the C5 and C6 vertebrae, travels to the upper biceps muscle, continues down to the forearm, and across the wrist to the thumb, index finger, and third finger. The C6 nerve terminates at the median nerve, which is the same nerve that can be compressed at the wrist and cause carpal tunnel syndrome. Therefore, if there is pain and tingling traveling down the forearm, across the wrist and into the fingers, it may be difficult to tell if the problem is due to carpal tunnel syndrome, C6 nerve injury, or both. With significant C6 nerve root injury, you may notice weakness in your biceps muscle, or when you try to bend the wrist back, or move your thumb.

The C7 nerve root exits the spine from in between C6 and C7, and is the motor nerve for the triceps and the wrist flexor muscles. The C7 nerve ends in the middle finger. The C8 nerve root exits between the C7 and C8 vertebrae. It travels down the inside of the forearm and ends in the last two fingers. It is partly responsible for the muscles of the hand that help make a fist.

OTHER PAIN PATTERNS

It can be confusing when pain due to a neck problem is felt in the upper back, shoulders, head, or face. Pain that is felt in an area remote from the site of injury or disease and not due to nerve compression is called referred pain. Referred pain is common in many medical and orthopedic conditions, and is discussed in chapter 2.

Pain in the shoulder area can be confusing, because it may be difficult to tell if the pain is due to a shoulder problem (such as rotator cuff tendinitis), a neck problem, or both. The neck and shoulder may have been hurt at the same time, or the shoulder may have been injured by being overworked while compensating for the neck problem. Referred pain felt between the shoulder blades is usually coming from the lower neck, but can also occasionally be due to a thoracic disc injury.

Neck injuries can cause pain that extends to the base of the skull and results in headache (see chapter 6). Some patients may also get headache behind an eye. When significant headache accompanies neck pain, this usually means that one or more of the upper three segments of the neck are the source of the pain. Injury to the upper two or three neck segments can also cause pain in the face.

Other Symptoms

Other symptoms that may be associated with neck problems include nausea, vomiting, dizziness, memory problems, difficulty concentrating, blurry vision, or depression. If any of these symptoms is present, it is important to discuss them with your doctor to be sure there are no other medical illnesses coexisting with the neck problem. However, fever is not associated with neck pain due to a structural problem, but can be

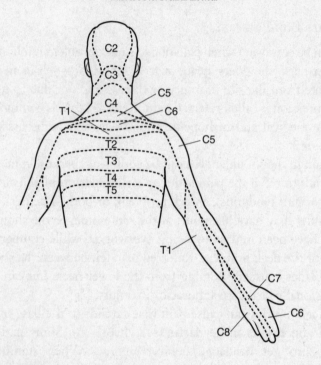

Figures 7 and 8
Dermatome charts of the upper body showing the distribution of nerves to the skin and muscles of the neck, upper back, and arms. Figure 7: Rear view. Figure 8: Front view.

due to an underlying infection or other medical problem. On rare occasions, large bone spurs may form in the front of discs and cause difficulty swallowing.

PHYSICAL EXAMINATION

The physical examination must always be interpreted with the patient's history in mind. By examining the patient, a doctor usually can determine if there is evidence of nerve dam-

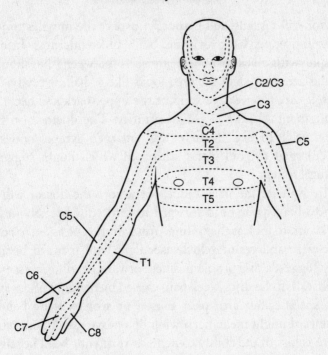

age, spinal cord compression, or medical causes for the neck pain.

The examination starts with inspection of the patient's posture, especially sitting posture. Many people with neck pain sit in a slumped position. The spine functions as a unit, so when your low back is not straight, you will tend to round your upper back and push your head and neck forward. This posture places abnormal mechanical stresses on the muscles, ligaments, discs, and facet joints of the neck. When I see that a patient has poor posture during my interview, I must assume they have poor posture during their usual activities of daily living.

During the physical exam, your doctor will inspect your skin to see whether you have shingles or a rash (see chapter 2). The doctor will visually and manually inspect the muscles of your neck and upper back for tone, bulk, and tenderness. In most people with neck pain, the muscles between the shoulder blades are small, and the area looks like a shallow cavity. The muscles are too weak to support the upper back and neck, and strengthening them is a high priority. The doctor also feels your neck to see if there are enlarged lymph nodes or an enlarged thyroid gland, either of which might suggest a medical illness.

To evaluate the neck range of motion, the doctor will ask you to bend your head forward toward your breastbone and backward to look at the ceiling. You will then be asked to rotate clockwise and counterclockwise. Pain with forward bending may suggest a disc problem, since forward bending stresses the back wall of the disc. Neck pain caused by bending backward is less specific, but arm pain caused or worsened by bending backward might mean narrowing of a nerve canal. Sometimes, there is loss of the ability to bend or turn your head because it hurts to do so. This type of finding does not help the doctor to tell where the pain is coming from, but it does tell about your ability to function.

Nerve root compression can cause muscle weakness, so your doctor will test your muscle strength. We are able to test the strength of the muscles supplied by C5, C6, C7, and C8 nerves (table 1). However, because many muscles receive more than one nerve and many nerves go to more than one muscle, strength testing is not totally specific.

When a nerve is compressed, it may decrease the reflex that is conducted along that particular nerve. Your doctor will check your reflexes by tapping the tendons and see if the muscle contracts. The reflexes and the nerves that serve them are shown in table 2. The most important reflexes are at the inside of the elbow (biceps, C5 and perhaps C6), the outside of the

Table 1

Nerve Supply and Functions of the Major Muscles

Nerve	Major Muscle	Muscle Action
C5	Deltoid	Lifting arms away from the sides of the body
C6	Biceps	"Making a muscle"; bringing forearm toward the chest
C7	Triceps	Pushing the bent forearm away from the chest
C8	Between the fingers	Spreading the fingers apart

elbow (triceps, C7), and thumb side of the forearm (brachiora-dialis, C6). Reflexes are graded on a scale of 0 (absent) to 4 (markedly increased). Each reflex is graded and also compared to the one on the other side. Side-to-side differences are usually most indicative of nerve root compression.

Table 2

Reflexes of the Major Cervical Nerves

Nerve	Reflex	Location
C5	Biceps	Inner elbow
C6	Biceps, forearm	Inner elbow and thumb side of the forearm
C7	Triceps	Outer elbow near the "funny bone"
C8	None	

If there is pressure on the spinal cord, the reflexes actually may be increased, and several abnormal reflexes may appear.

One abnormal reflex is called Hoffmann's sign. When the nail is "flicked," the thumb moves. Another abnormal reflex is called clonus. When the foot is rapidly forced up toward the shin, the ankle jerks repeatedly. These reflexes, although sometimes indicating pressure on the spinal cord, also can be normal in a small number of people, so they must be interpreted in conjunction with the history, remainder of the examination, and diagnostic tests.

Sensory tests are done to look for partial or complete numbness along the route of a particular nerve or, in cases of neuropathy, many small nerves (figures 7 and 8). To evaluate sensation, your doctor will stroke your skin with his or her fingers, a clean safety pin, or a light brush. In the past, doctors used a pinwheel, but because it is sharp, and can break the skin, there is a danger of transmitting a virus or other infection. Therefore, it should no longer be used.

Your doctor will also examine your shoulders to check for bursitis, tendinitis, or joint problems. He or she will examine the nerves that go through the bones at each wrist to check for carpal tunnel syndrome, and the nerve at each elbow to see if the ulnar nerve is being compressed at the area of the "funny bone." Your head may be pushed down, rotated, or stretched to look for disc herniation. There are additional tests that can be performed as well, and the exam I described is a minimum exam. If your doctor suspects other problems, he or she may do other tests during the examination.

DIAGNOSTIC TESTS

There are many diagnostic tests that may help determine the cause of neck pain, including X-rays, magnetic resonance imaging scan (MRI), computed tomography scan (CT), electrical nerve studies (EMG/NCV), myelogram, and spinal injections. The choice and timing of testing vary according to the severity of pain, duration of the pain, clinical suspicions of the doctor, and the findings on your physical examination. Most patients will not need any tests because the pain gets better with treatment. However, patients who do not improve and those with significant abnormalities on physical examination may require testing.

X-rays

Plain X-rays can play a role in the diagnosis of cervical spine problems. X-rays only show bone; they do not show discs or soft tissues. X-rays are not useful initially in neck pain, but become important when a patient is not responding to conservative care after several months.

When indicated, neck X-rays should include a front view and side views with the patient bending the head forward (flexion) and backward (extension). A narrowed disc space indicates that a disc has worn down, and might be the source of pain. Although a narrowed disc space takes many years to develop, these worn discs are more susceptible to acute injury such as after a car accident. Bone spurs indicate more advanced disc degeneration, and although not visible on plain X-ray, if bone spurs have grown into the nerve canal, they may compress the nerve.

X-rays may show a loss of the normal spinal curve. This is usually interpreted to mean there is muscle spasm, but it may also mean there is a disc injury at the level where the curve flattens out or changes direction. The flexion and extension views may pinpoint a single level that does not move as well as the other levels (which suggests an injury at that level), or may disclose too much motion (instability), which can cause pain.

Magnetic Resonance Imaging (MRI)

MRI scan is one of the most useful tests for neck problems. MRI scans have replaced myelograms in most spine centers, although there are some doctors who still prefer myelograms (see page 57). MRI uses a magnetic field and radio waves to produce a picture of the spine. It shows discs, the spinal cord, spinal fluid sac (thecal sac), spinal nerves, and the surrounding soft tissues directly, but does not show bone. The MRI does not use X-rays or radiation, so it is extremely safe. The patient lies in a closed tube, so some people with claustrophobia may require a mild sedative to get through the test. There are also "open scanners" that are far less claustrophobic, but the image quality is not usually quite as good because the open MRI scanners must use a weaker magnet, and the best images are obtained by a scanner with a magnet of 1.5 Tesla.

The most frequent reason for ordering an MRI is to examine the discs, nerve roots, and spinal cord. Disc injuries can cause pain when a herniated disc presses against a nerve or the spinal cord, or when the wall of a disc has been torn, all of which are usually visible on MRI. The MRI also will reveal infections, tumors, and other medical problems in the neck.

MRI should be performed on an urgent basis when there is evidence on physical examination of a compressed spinal cord, pressure on a major nerve root, or if infection or cancer is suspected. In other situations, MRI is indicated if a patient is not getting better after three or four months of treatment, and there is need for a definite diagnosis. MRI is also indicated when cervical spine injections are being considered (see page 59), or when pain is severe enough that surgery is being considered.

Computerized Tomography (CT Scan or CAT Scan)

Computerized tomography is more commonly called CT scan or CAT scan. CT scans use X-rays to produce pictures of the spine. Although there is some radiation, CT scans are extremely safe. The scanner is open, and therefore does not usually cause a feeling of claustrophobia. CT scan does not show soft tissues as well as an MRI does, but provides a direct view of the bones and the nerve canals. To obtain the best imaging quality, the CT should provide pictures in three planes, side to side, front to back, and top to bottom. CT is sometimes done immediately after a myelogram or discogram to augment the information from these tests.

CT can be useful to evaluate patients with prior neck fusions to see if the fusion appears solid. It also is valuable in patients who cannot tolerate an MRI. CT will show disc herniations well, but does not show the interior of the disc.

Myelogram

Many years ago, myelogram was the only test available to view the inside of the spinal canal, but compared with the more modern MRI and CT scans, it gives a much less detailed view of the anatomy of the spinal cord and nerves. When CT scan was first used to evaluate neck pain, it was often done immediately after a myelogram to increase the information. When MRI scans became available, they eliminated the need for myelogram for most patients. However, some doctors who were trained in the myelogram era still rely on this test.

A myelogram is an X-ray technique. A liquid that shows up well on X-ray is injected into the spinal cord sac and X-rays are taken. The liquid outlines the nerve structures and the radiologist looks for indentations or blockages of the "dye" column that may indicate bone spurs or disc herniations. There are limitations and disadvantages to this test. For example, a myelogram tells us nothing about the internal architecture of the disc, nor does it show the lateral spinal canals well. In addition, the myelogram is invasive. It requires an injection, and may cause a headache that can last for several days.

Electromyography (EMG) and Nerve Conduction Velocity (NCV)

The radiological tests described above allow us to obtain pictures of anatomy, but do not tell us anything about physiology. When it is necessary to know if there is nerve damage, EMG (electromyography) and NCV (nerve conduction velocity) can provide useful information. Many patients have pain, but no nerve damage. Therefore, EMG and NCV must be interpreted in conjunction with the history, examination, MRI, and clinical suspicions. The EMG and NCV can determine if there is nerve damage, which nerves are damaged, if the damage is acute or chronic, and if the problem is due to injury at the elbow or wrist.

Several of the nerves that originate in the neck travel down to the arm, wrist, and hands, and therefore a nerve can be damaged at several sites along its path. For example, the C6 nerve becomes the median nerve, which travels to the hand through the carpal tunnel at the wrist. Therefore, pain, numbness, weakness, or tingling in the hand in a C6 distribution can come from nerve injury in the neck, the wrist, or both. The C7 nerve travels behind the elbow, and can be compressed at the "funny bone" or occasionally in the wrist. The EMG and

NCV can distinguish between nerve damage in the neck, elbow, or wrist.

Nerves can also be damaged by medical diseases such as diabetes or alcoholism. This type of damage is called peripheral neuropathy, and will be apparent on NCV.

To perform an EMG, the doctor inserts very fine needles that are attached to wires and to an oscilloscope into specific muscles. The patient will feel a slight prick from the needle and then a tingling sensation as a very small amount of current is applied. It is only slightly painful, and not at all dangerous.

Diagnostic Injections

MEDIAL BRANCH BLOCKS (MBB)

Facet joints can be a cause of neck pain in at least 15 percent of people with neck pain and up to 40 percent of patients with whiplash. There is no correlation between the appearance of a facet joint on X-ray or CT scan and whether the joint is painful. Facet joints receive their nerve supplies from the medial branch of the dorsal ramus of the spinal nerve (called medial branch for short). Each joint actually receives medial branches from two separate spinal nerves. Therefore, to determine if a joint is a source of pain, it is necessary to anesthetize both nerves by placing local anesthetic around them. If there is pain relief immediately after the injection, it is good evidence that the joint was causing the pain. If there is no relief, it eliminates the joint from consideration as a source of pain. Frequently, more than one joint may be involved, so all suspicious joints must be tested.

The procedure causes minimal pain and is very safe. However, it should be done under fluoroscopic visual guidance. It is much less useful to inject the joint itself, because the joint may leak and the local anesthetic spill over out onto the nerve root. If this occurs, there may be pain relief, but for the wrong reason.

If it can be proven that one or more facet joint is the source of the pain, it can be treated quite effectively by a technique called radiofrequency neurotomy. An insulated needle connected to a radiofrequency generator is placed on the nerve. The needle is heated to coagulate the nerve, which then can no longer conduct pain signals. The improvement usually lasts six to eighteen months, and when pain recurs, the procedure can be repeated.

SELECTIVE NERVE ROOT BLOCK (SNRB)

Selective nerve root injection might also be called transforaminal epidural. It can provide both diagnostic information and pain relief, particularly relief of arm pain due to herniated disc or narrowing of a nerve root canal. In the SNRB, the area around a single nerve is injected with a local anesthetic and corticosteroid. In patients with disc herniation, some patients can avoid surgery with a series of SNRBs.

DISCOGRAPHY

Discography is a test in which discs are injected in order to pressurize them and thereby determine if they are causing the neck pain. It is used only when there is persistent and severe neck pain that has not responded to conservative treatment, and surgery is being considered. It is not a routine test, and it is somewhat controversial. Some spine specialists use it routinely to plan possible surgery, but others feel it has no role in the evaluation of neck pain or the planning of surgery.

Discography should be done by a physician experienced in performing this procedure. Under X-ray imaging, the physician inserts a needle into the center of the disc. The disc is then slowly injected with a radiological contrast medium (sometimes called "dye"). The most important part of the test is the pain response. A normal disc barely hurts, but injecting a disc that is contributing to the pain will reproduce the patient's pain. At least three discs should be tested, because it is important to find a painless disc to serve as a control, or comparison, to those that are painful. An X-ray is taken after the injections are completed to see the anatomy of the inside of the disc, but, once again, it is the pain provocation part of the test that is most important.

Cervical discography has been utilized to evaluate cervical discs since 1957. My colleagues and I reviewed our experience with cervical discography to determine the complication rate. We found that discography performed by a very experienced physician is extremely safe. In addition, we found that occasionally a disc that appears normal on MRI can be the source of neck pain, and discs that appear abnormal on MRI may be painless on discography.

4
Whiplash and Whiplash-Associated Disorders

Whiplash has a very negative public image. The mere mention of the term brings up an image of a person with a neck brace who is exaggerating his or her symptoms in anticipation of a big legal settlement. Some people think that everyone with whiplash is "faking it," or at least embellishing the symptoms. Although there are some individuals who try to take advantage of any situation, even a car accident, whiplash is very real, and it is responsible for a great deal of pain, suffering, and disability.

The term "whiplash" can be confusing because it describes both a mechanism of injury and the symptoms caused by an injury. The mechanism of injury is any incident that causes the head and neck to move suddenly and forcefully in one direction and then recoil ("whip") in the opposite direction. In a rear-end-impact car accident, the upper body is thrust forward, leaving the head and neck behind, which in essence forces the head and neck backward. In addition, the upper body moves upward, which causes the neck to form an unnatural S-shape

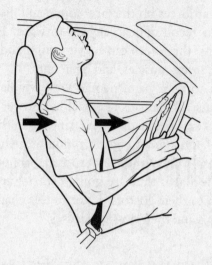

Figures 9 and 10

Whiplash mechanics. Figure 9: In a rear-end collision, the upper body is thrust forward, but the head lags behind. Figure 10: Almost instantly, the head and neck then "whip" forward to catch up to the upper body.

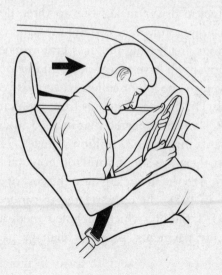

and places great forces on the facet joints and discs. The head and neck then recoil and accelerate forward. Even in low-speed collisions, the forces can be very high and sufficient to damage joints, discs, muscles, and ligaments.

In addition to neck pain, people with whiplash may have other symptoms. Their arms may feel heavy, weak, or painful. They may also experience dizziness, ringing in the ears, visual disturbances, fatigue, poor concentration or memory, and difficulty sleeping. When these unexpected symptoms persist, patients may feel as if they are going "crazy," and hesitate to mention them to their doctors. Later in this chapter, I discuss these symptoms and their possible causes.

WHIPLASH FACTS AND FIGURES

To understand why whiplash has become so common, it is important to review some facts and figures about automobile accidents. Driving has become very challenging. According to Dr. Lawrence Nordhoff, author of the 1996 *Motor Vehicle Crash Injuries*, the typical driver makes one to three decisions each second, at least one error every two minutes, and crosses 1 million intersections in a driving life. It is little wonder, then, that the average driver will have a near-accident one or two times a month and average one minor collision every six years.

In his book, Dr. Nordhoff quotes from the National Safety Council (NSC), which reported that in 1993, there were 11.9 million accidents involving 21 million vehicles. The NSC also estimated that there are about 5 million nonfatal injuries each year. In addition to the medical issues, the cost of car accidents is staggering. In 1988, the costs related to car accidents were more than $333 billion, which included medical costs, lost wages, disability payments, property damage payments, and legal fees.

Most people think they are excellent drivers, and it is always the other drivers who do stupid, careless, or dangerous things. Most drivers feel they are in complete control over their cars and can afford to take a few chances. Some accidents are caused by drivers who are overconfident about their skills, and their abilities to anticipate road conditions and other drivers' reactions. There are some factors that are under our control and play a role in accidents. Risky driving, especially by inexperienced drivers, and a stubborn failure to yield add to the chances of a car accident. Inattention while driving, especially when speaking on a cellular phone, is an increasingly common cause of accidents. Medical problems, such as poor and uncorrected vision and some chronic illnesses, may play a role in increased accidents, as does sleep deprivation. Finally, the use of alcohol or illicit drugs before or while driving is very dangerous.

MECHANICS OF WHIPLASH

Many physicians and attorneys believe the primary reason whiplash patients continue to have pain is the potential for financial gains from a lawsuit. They may not appreciate the large magnitude of the forces delivered to the head and neck in even a low-speed collision. However, scientists who study whiplash have published their findings in scientific journals and have shown that significant and long-lasting neck pain is very real, very common, and readily explained. Even the most cynical doctors and lawyers should admit that not everyone with neck pain after low-speed accidents can be faking. To appreciate how seemingly minor impacts can cause major problems, it is necessary to understand a few simple concepts of physics—change in velocity, expressed as delta-V, and change in acceleration, expressed as G forces.

Change in velocity is essentially the change in speed. For example, if a stopped car is hit from behind by a second car (called the bullet vehicle) of equal weight and traveling at 10 miles per hour (mph), the first car will be knocked forward. Almost instantly, its speed will change from 0 mph (stopped) to about 5 mph—roughly one-half the speed of the vehicle that struck it. If the bullet vehicle weighs significantly more than the first car, or if it is traveling faster than 10 mph at impact, the delta-V of the struck car will be even greater. Delta-V is one of the factors that determine the forces placed on the car and its occupants.

"Acceleration" is the term used to describe how fast this change in velocity occurs, and it is expressed in Gs. One G is the force of gravity; ten Gs would be ten times the force of gravity. Jet pilots use Gs to describe the pressure that forces them back against their seats when the plane takes off or when it accelerates in midflight. If the velocity of a car changes from 0 mph to 5 mph in one minute, acceleration is slow and the G forces are low. On the other hand, if a car goes from 0 mph to 5 mph in one-tenth of a second, acceleration is rapid, and G forces are high. The higher the Gs, the greater the forces placed on the heads and necks of the car's occupants.

When a vehicle is hit from the rear, the forces are transmitted very rapidly from the bullet vehicle to the struck car and its occupants. Injury to the neck occurs due to a combination of extension, compression, shear forces, and recoil.

In a rear-end impact, the body does not move as one single unit. Instead, the torso, base of the neck, and upper neck move somewhat separately. Within one-tenth of a second after impact, the impact energy is transferred from the frame of the car to the car seat and then to the torso of the occupant. The forward motion of the car seat pushes the torso forward and upward, but the head and neck lag behind. The forward movement of the torso places the neck into extension in relation to the torso, and the upward movement compresses the cervical region from below. Approximately six-hundredths of a second later, the base (lowest part) of the neck begins to move forward to "catch up" to the torso, which produces a shearing action. The combined movements place large forces on the facet joints and discs, and is one of the major causes of whiplash injury.

The torso continues to move forward while the neck lags behind. The neck is forced into more extension, which may cause further damage to the facet joints and the discs. Finally, in order for the head and upper neck to "catch up" to the torso, they accelerate forward ("whip") rapidly, which produces very high G forces on the neck with the potential for further damage.

The forces at the top of the head can reach seventeen Gs in a 9 mph rear-end accident! The average head weighs about ten pounds. Therefore, in a low-speed accident, the forces placed on the top of the neck at maximum acceleration can be as high as 170 pounds (seventeen Gs times ten pounds)! Because of the shape of the neck, most of the energy is absorbed at the C5 to C7 area, and the C1 to C3 region suffers the next highest forces.

These facts of physics and biomechanics demonstrate how low-speed collisions can subject the neck to powerful forces and cause significant damage to the ligaments, discs, and joints. At higher speeds, the incidence of whiplash injury is greater. At impact speeds of 5 mph, the incidence of neck injuries may be 10 percent, but at impact speeds of 10 mph, the incidence of whiplash may be as high as 45 percent!

In addition to the speeds of the vehicles, there are other factors that contribute to whiplash injuries. These include use of shoulder and lap restraints, head restraint type and position, direction of impact, and the human factors.

Seat Belts

The use of seat belts also affects the frequency of neck pain after an accident. While the use of three-point shoulder and lap restraints has markedly reduced the fatality rate from car accidents, the lower death rate has come at a price. There has been a 26 percent increase in whiplash injury since the introduction of lap belts, and a 31 percent increase since the use of shoulder and lap restraints.

Head Restraints

The position and type of the head restraint (also incorrectly called headrest) plays a role in neck injuries. The head restraint is designed to keep the head and neck aligned with the upper body at impact, which would decrease the chances of injury. The head and neck would not lag so far behind the torso and so would not be forced into extension, nor would the head and neck be whipped forward. The head restraint is meant to work as a restraint, not a headrest. It should be positioned high enough so it is in contact with the back of the head. There is an increased frequency of neck pain after car accidents if the headrest is too low.

Head restraints can be fixed or adjustable. Fixed restraints are the most effective, and can reduce neck injuries by 25 percent. Adjustable restraints are less effective, but still reduce the frequency of neck injuries by about 15 percent. Adjustable restraints are not as effective for the following reasons:

• Incorrect usage and position: Some drivers feel the lowered position looks better and does not block their vision. Clearly, though, the potential for whiplash increases if the restraint is not positioned high enough to restrain the back of the head.

- Construction of the adjustable restraints: Adjustable head restraints sit on vertical metal supports that flex on impact and then recoil slightly, adding to the whiplash effect. Manufacturers who emphasize safety over cosmetics usually install fixed head restraints.

Direction of Impact

The direction the vehicles are moving at the time of the crash plays a role in the type of injury. One research study of neck pain after motor vehicle accidents showed that the incidence of neck pain was 31 percent after rear-impact collisions, 23 percent after frontal collisions, 17 percent after right-side collisions, and 11 percent after left-side collisions. Those in the rear seat had only one-half the incidence of neck pain of those seated in the front. There is also an increased incidence of neck injuries if the person's head strikes the windshield.

If the occupant's head is turned, there may also be an increase in the incidence and severity of the neck injury.

Human Factors

Some people are more vulnerable to injury than others. There are wide variations in body sizes, shapes, muscle tone, and pain tolerances. Some people have discs or joints that have been weakened from prior injuries, poor posture, or chronic overuse, and are more susceptible to whiplash injury. Many of these factors are out of our control, but they still affect the outcome of a motor vehicle accident.

Whiplash: The Onset of Pain

Most people with whiplash begin to have pain within twenty-four hours of their car accidents, but it is not unusual for pain to begin later. After any trauma, powerful hormones that reduce pain—called endorphins—may be released. In addition, in response to the stress of the accident, other biochemicals, such as adrenaline, are released to prepare the body for "fight or flight" and may also reduce pain. After a few days, when the levels of these hormones drop, pain that was temporarily suppressed occurs.

Some of the pain after whiplash may be due to inflammation. Because it may take several days for inflammation to set in, there may be a delay before the onset of pain. This is similar to a sprained ankle. Although there may be some pain immediately after an ankle sprain, it is common for the pain to increase over the next twenty-four to forty-eight hours as inflammation takes hold. There is recent research that shows that administering powerful medications called steroids soon after an accident will lower the incidence of chronic neck pain, because these drugs prevent much of the inflammation.

Whiplash: The Possible Causes of the Pain

In most patients with neck pain due to a car accident, it is not necessary to know the cause of the pain because initial treatment is straightforward and improvement is usually rapid. However, for those patients who do not get better after six months or so, and who have no specific findings on examination or tests, there may be confusion. Their doctors may not know what is wrong, their insurance companies and its lawyers think nothing is wrong, the patients' attorneys think everything is wrong, and the patients begin to think they are crazy.

Whiplash specialists have learned a great deal about the causes of neck pain, and what to do when the usual test results are normal but symptoms persist. Unfortunately, this newer information has not yet reached the general medical and legal communities, which may result in incorrect diagnoses, inadequate treatment, and unnecessarily large legal expenses.

In the first few weeks to months after a motor vehicle accident , it is preferable to refer to the pain as "nonspecific neck pain," which is a better term than muscle strain, muscle sprain, or soft tissue injury. We know the muscles and ligaments have been strained and are probably inflamed, but these soft tissues should heal within three to four months. Pain that remains is usually due to other problems.

Neck pain that is still present after four months usually is due to injuries to the facet joints, the discs, or both (see chapters 2 and 3). In several research studies of whiplash patients, the facet joints have been shown to be the major cause of neck pain in more than one-half of patients. Other scientists have shown that 23 percent of the time, the facet joints were the sole cause of pain; that 20 percent of the time discs were the only cause of pain; and that 41 percent of the time both the facet joints and discs were responsible for the pain. In only 17 percent of patients the cause of the pain was not determined.

WHIPLASH-ASSOCIATED SYMPTOMS

Whiplash patients sometimes can have unusual complaints, and doctors may label these symptoms as being psychologically based. However, since so many patients experience such similar symptoms after whiplash, it is very likely that there is a physical reason for them, even if they are not readily explained. Many complain of headaches, pain in the shoulders, pain between the shoulder blades, or arm pains. Neck-related headaches (see chapter 6) are usually located at the base of the skull, the crown of the head, the forehead, or the face and jaw. They are often due to injuries to the upper cervical facet joints or discs.

Pain in the shoulders, between the shoulder blades, or in the arms can be due to direct pressure on nerves but is more likely to be referred from other structures in the neck. "Referred pain" is pain that is felt at a location away from the diseased or injured areas, but not due to a compressed nerve (see chapter 2). It is often poorly localized, at least partly because it does not follow the path of a single nerve. In addition to pain, whiplash patients may feel tired or dizzy. Some notice poor concentration, memory problems, or difficulty sleeping. Others are irritable, depressed, or short-tempered. There may be blurry vision, ringing in the ears, or a feeling of heaviness in the arms.

About one-third of patients with whiplash have problems with concentration or memory. Sometimes, patients are hesitant to mention these types of problems because they feel ashamed. However, it is important to report them to the doctor because they may be symptoms of other problems, many of which require specific treatment. There are several possible reasons for these problems. The pain itself can be a great distraction, depression may cause difficulties with concentration, and medications such as muscle relaxants, sedatives, and narcotics used to treat the pain can affect thinking and emotions.

One very important cause of changes in emotions or thinking is a minor injury to the brain from the whiplash, which is called traumatic brain injury or postconcussion syndrome. Traumatic brain injury occurs because the brain is soft and the skull is hard. When the head and neck are "whipped" forward, the brain continues to move after the skull has already stopped. The soft brain strikes the inside of the hard skull. There does not need to be a loss of consciousness, and some do not even have a headache right away. In these cases, an MRI and CAT scans of the brain are usually normal, but specialized neuro-psychological tests will disclose the effects of the brain injury.

It is critical to diagnose brain injury for several reasons. Most important, if treatment is begun within the first six to twelve months, there is a much greater chance things will get better. Secondly, once the patient and family understand that there is a physical basis for the changes in personality and thinking, they feel a great sense of relief. In addition, in my experience, pain in patients with brain injury takes longer to get better than in other whiplash patients. Patients with brain injury may take longer to learn the exercises and body mechanics, and often need to have even simple instructions repeated many times. There are also social and economic problems. Some patients may not be able to return to their old jobs because of the mental changes, even if the pain is better. Therefore, diagnosis of these problems early can allow the family to access specialized resources to plan for the future and help with the recovery.

Many patients with whiplash also have low back pain. Most likely, the low back pain is due to an injury to this area at the same time as the neck was injured, rather than that the neck problem is causing the back pain. Sitting produces the greatest mechanical stresses on the low back, and when a car is hit from the rear, the car seat back flexes forward while the hips are held in place by the seat belt. These opposing forces can injure the discs or joints of the low back.

WHIPLASH: THE LONG-TERM OUTCOME

I have already stated several times that most people with neck pain due to a car accident recover quickly and completely,

although there is great variation in the rate of healing. There
are dozens of scientific research articles that have evaluated the
rates of recovery from whiplash, and virtually all have come to
the same conclusions. After three to four weeks, most people
are better, but it is very common for symptoms to last for three
or four months, and occasionally longer. However, by six
months after an accident, most patients who are going to get
completely better will already be well, and by one year, 80 percent or 90 percent of patients who are going to get better will
be fully recovered. The remaining 10 percent to 20 percent of
patients have chronic neck pain, and these are the patients who
pose the greatest challenges to the medical, legal, and insurance
systems. The subject of whiplash and the legal system is discussed in detail in the next chapter.

Some readers may be interested in one example of the
research about the outcome of whiplash. One group of
researchers treated 117 whiplash patients for several years. By
three months, 66 percent of their patients had recovered; by six
months, 70 percent had recovered; by twelve months, 76 percent had recovered; and by twenty-four months, 82 percent
had recovered. After six months, the rate of further recovery
was very slow. Even with expert treatment, 18 percent of their
patients had significant pain two years after the accident! If
prior to the accident there was neck pain, arthritis in the neck,
or headaches, the prognosis was not as good. In addition, pain
that began right after the accident, older age, or head rotated
to either side at the time of impact were factors that put the
patients at higher risk for poor outcome.

Other scientists have estimated the impact of chronic neck
pain due to whiplash in the general population. If it is assumed
there is one case of whiplash for every one thousand people, 25
percent of people with whiplash develop chronic neck pain, the

average age of a whiplash patient is thirty, with a life expectancy of seventy, there would be 1 percent of the population with chronic neck pain after a whiplash injury! In one-third of these people, the pain would be severe. You can see how whiplash is an extraordinary problem!

5
Whiplash and the Legal System

In our litigious society, many people who have neck pain due to a car accident file lawsuits to attempt to retrieve money spent on car repairs, medical bills, lost wages, and to ask for compensation for their pain and suffering. Our society has come to view those who bring lawsuits (plaintiffs) in accident cases as profit seekers.

In this chapter, I will discuss the factors that contribute to this perception, and the ways in which science is used and interpreted by both plaintiff and defense attorneys in lawsuits involving whiplash. Although we might think that the potential for financial gain from a lawsuit would unconsciously make an accident victim's pain and disability worse, there is no good scientific evidence to support this idea. Physicians, attorneys, and insurers should not make decisions or render medical-legal opinions based on preexisting ideas—they should rely on scientific evidence. However, in many cases, the legal system has not caught up with current medical research. In addition, many others besides the injured parties have their own incentives for being involved in accident cases. Therefore, it should prove informative to look at the facts about lawsuits and whiplash.

The "Business" of Accidents

Often the accident victim is singled out as the one who is trying to profit by filing suit, but it is not just the whiplash patient who stands to benefit financially from a motor vehicle accident. In fact, car accidents and injuries constitute a multi-million-dollar industry in the United States. The most obvious businesses that profit are the auto repair shops that make money fixing damaged cars. Physicians, chiropractors, and physical therapists are paid to treat the injured party. In addition, some doctors earn a substantial portion of their incomes by doing "independent" medical evaluations and testifying as expert witnesses. Their future referrals may depend on their opinions and performances in deposition and at trial.

Lawyers also earn money from accidents. Attorneys for accident victims (called plaintiff's attorneys) usually work on a contingency basis, which means they only get paid if they win the case. On the other hand, most defense attorneys get paid by the hour, which could work as an incentive to "drag things out a bit." Engineers, called accident reconstructionists, are paid to figure out the forces at impact, and then determine whether the forces were great enough to cause injuries. In some cases, economists are hired to testify about potential lost earnings. Even jurors receive small payments to serve on a jury panel, and if they are government employees, they are paid their full salaries while serving. Insurance companies sell insurance, and profits are greater if losses are less. It is a tangled financial web, with each accident creating its own little industry.

Medical Science and the Legal System

Several legal issues apply to physicians involved with personal injury lawsuits. Doctors are supposed to practice "evidence-based medicine," which means that their diagnoses, treatments, and opinions should be based on scientific evidence, not personal beliefs or biases. The most current information is available to all doctors because it is published in medical journals, described in textbooks, discussed at medical meetings, and available via the Internet. The field of medicine changes quickly, and doctors must work hard to stay current. This is no different in the field of whiplash, where there has been so much information published in the last few years. The next sections outline the ways in which scientific evidence is used by the respective sides in personal injury cases.

"Independent" Medical Evaluations

In our adversarial legal system, each side must argue that their interpretation of the facts is the correct one. In personal injury suits, both the plaintiff and the insurance company hire attorneys. In order to help clarify the medical aspects of a whiplash case, each attorney obtains a medical opinion from a physician about the cause of the patient's pain, his or her diagnosis, future needs for medical care, and disability, if any. Although the doctor is supposed to be unbiased and "independent," this may not always be true. Attorneys usually hire doctors with whom they have worked in the past, and who have offered them advantageous opinions. Some of these doctors earn a large portion of their incomes doing independent medical evaluations and many work exclusively for one side or the other. Their future work may depend on their current and past opinions. Finally, doctors who see a patient only once have no responsibility to see or treat the patient again. After the case is over, they never have to explain their opinions to the patient or look the patient in the eye again.

There are no strict guidelines for a doctor to be qualified as an "expert." It is up to a judge to decide if a doctor qualifies as an expert and a jury to decide which expert is better qualified and offers the best opinion. With respect to neck pain, defense attorneys usually employ orthopedic surgeons, neurosurgeons, or neurologists. However, a doctor's specialty does not automatically determine his or her level of expertise. Orthopedists and neurosurgeons are trained primarily in hospitals, and learn their skills treating seriously ill patients. During training, it may be rare for them to see office patients with neck pain after car accidents. In the hospital, they treat patients with neck fractures or those that are there for surgery. During training, they do not spend much time in doctors' offices, where most patients with neck pain are seen. As a result, they may not have been trained to thoroughly evaluate and treat patients with neck pain who do not require surgery. They may even have developed the opinion that if a patient's condition is not bad enough to need surgery, there may really be nothing wrong. Just because doctors are neurosurgeons or orthopedic surgeons, that does not mean they are truly experts, especially since it is the rare whiplash patient who needs surgery.

Some attorneys use neurologists as experts. Neurologists are trained to evaluate and treat patients with nerve injuries or diseases, not patients with bone, joint, disc, or even soft tissue problems. One opinion holds that because the patient complains of pain, and pain involves nerves, then a neurologist is best suited to be an expert witness. However, no attorney would claim that a neurologist should be used as an expert with a patient with chest pain or stomach pain. Instead, a cardiologist or gastroenterologist would be the appropriate choice of expert specialist.

The best experts, therefore, should be doctors who devote a significant portion of their practices and much of their continuing education to the spine. They should be doctors who treat patients on a regular basis, rather than those who just offer legal opinions. Proper educational background ideally would include specialty training or years of clinical experience treating patients with spine problems. To keep up to date, they should read specialty journals about disorders of the spine and attend specialty meetings devoted to the spine. Membership in professional societies that offer continuing education about the spine, such as the North American Spine Society, would also be desirable. In addition, the highest level of experts are those who are teaching medical students, residents, or fellows; writing articles; and performing research about spine problems.

In some cases, plaintiff attorneys may not need to hire independent medical examiners, because they can rely on the patient's treating doctor. However, treating doctors may have their own biases. They may know their patients and their families well, because they have seen them several times. They will probably continue to see their patients after their cases have been settled, and so must maintain a trusting relationship.

Abnormal Magnetic Resonance Imaging (MRI) Scans

One example of how science can be used to support different sides of the same issue is the interpretation of MRI scans of the neck. MRI scanning is a sophisticated diagnostic tool, but the interpretation can be tricky. Findings on MRI do not tell us whether a person has pain. Some people can hurt and have normal MRIs, while others are pain free and have abnormal MRIs. Two recent scientific studies have shown that, depending on age, as many as 20 percent to 30 percent of people with no neck pain will have some evidence of disc changes on an MRI of the neck, and the percentage increases with advancing age. Some people even have herniated discs. Some attorneys and doctors may interpret this fact incorrectly, and use it to discount MRI findings. It is important to note that the patients in these studies did not have neck pain, so it is not correct science to apply these findings to people *with* neck pain.

It is also important to realize that while 20 percent to 30 percent of people without neck pain will have abnormal MRI scans, the remaining 70 percent to 80 percent of people without neck pain will have normal MRI scans. It is therefore much more likely that a person without neck pain will have a normal MRI. This suggests that when there are abnormal findings on MRI in a person with neck pain, it may indicate a cause for the pain.

Sometimes, MRI scans are read as normal because there is no disc herniation or compression of a nerve root or spinal cord, even though there may be some changes in the discs. This is because there is confusion regarding the concepts of normal and common. Normal means there are no structural changes on the scan—none. Common means that any structural changes present are seen frequently in others of the same age. Just because a finding is common does not mean it is nomal.

Neck Strain, Neck Sprain, and Myofascial Pain

Pinpointing the cause of neck pain may require a high level of expertise, and sophisticated diagnostic testing (see chapter 3), especially if the case is chronic. In litigated cases, certain diagnoses are very popular among independent medical experts employed by the defense. Perhaps the most common diagnosis used in these instances is "chronic neck sprain or strain." These diagnoses imply that there is no significant structural damage to deep structures, but there is a chronic injury to the muscles or ligaments of the neck that causes the pain. In fact, there are no scientific studies to show that chronic neck sprain or strain even exists. There are no objective ways to prove these diagnoses, and their mention usually indicates the doctor does not know the exact cause of the pain. These terms should be avoided, and when the diagnosis is not clear, it is preferable to use the term "neck pain, nonspecific."

Another popular diagnosis is myofascial pain. This diagnosis implies that pain is due to problems in the muscles or the fascia, a fibrous tissue that lies in between the muscles. Once again, there are no scientific studies to prove the diagnosis of myofascial pain exists. Even experts in muscle pain who examine the same patients do not agree on which muscles are the cause of the pain. In addition, the area of the tender muscles is usually right over a facet joint or other deeper structure, which makes it impossible to tell where tenderness is coming from. There are no findings on examination, X-ray, MRI scans, laboratory tests, or electrical nerve or muscle tests to confirm such a diagnosis.

A doctor who diagnoses neck strain or sprain would expect the patient to improve within four to six weeks, because most acute sprains or strains in other parts of the body get better over this period of time. When a patient does not get better, a doctor may attribute the chronic pain to psychological problems, faking, exaggerating, or an effect of the lawsuit, rather than considering the possibility that the diagnosis of strain or sprain is not correct.

Pain is invisible, and there are no tests that prove or disprove its existence. However, there are tests that show the anatomy of the neck. When we see abnormal findings on X-rays or MRI scans, and other tests, it is the job of the doctor to decide if the abnormalities on the tests are the cause of the patient's pain. It is unfortunate that some patients are given a diagnosis of sprain, strain, or myofascial pain (even though there are no objective tests to prove these diagnoses), while the objective abnormalities on X-ray or MRI are dismissed as normal. I have seen too many patients in whom an independent medical examiner made a diagnosis of sprain or strain despite a herniated disc visible on MRI and pain in the exact location expected from that particular disc herniation. At times, the examiner will go so far as to say the diagnosis is chronic strain and the disc herniation is an incidental finding!

Inadequate Knowledge of Disc or Facet Joint Pain

It has been proven that facet joint injury, disc injury, and combinations of disc and facet joint injuries are the most common causes of chronic neck pain after a car accident. This information has been studied by experts in the fields of spinal medicine, spine surgery, and pain management, and published in the medical journals. The information about how to make the correct diagnosis and how to treat such injuries is also available in the published medical literature. However, some doctors do not read these journals or attend the specialty meetings at which they are discussed. They rely instead on what they learned in medical school or in residency training. As a result, their diagnoses may be out-of-date.

The Role of Prior Neck Pain

Some patients with neck pain after a whiplash injury have had neck pain in the past. In some patients, the prior pain may have completely resolved, but others may have some degree of chronic neck pain at the time of the new accident. From a legal perspective, it is important to determine whether the new pain is totally due to the accident, partially due to the accident, or completely unrelated to the accident. Some scientific studies have addressed the importance of this problem. It has been proven that patients whose X-rays already show degenerative changes at the time of a new car accident are likely to have pain that is more severe and that lasts longer than patients with normal X-rays. This just means that people with previous neck injuries are more vulnerable to injury in a new accident.

Sometimes, lawyers refer to this condition of prior injury as a "thin shell," referring to the thickness of an eggshell. If an egg is dropped to the floor, it will probably break. The thinner the shell, the less distance it can fall before it breaks. Patients who have had prior neck pain probably have a "thin shell," and it takes less trauma to injure damaged discs than healthy ones.

SECONDARY GAIN AND MALINGERING

Secondary gain is an unconscious psychological process that refers to any advantages gained by a person as a consequence of his or her symptoms. In other words, a person achieves some benefit from neck pain that he or she could not get otherwise—benefits for feeling bad. There are many types of secondary gain, but the one that is of concern here is the potential for monetary gain from a lawsuit that arises from injuries sustained in a motor vehicle accident.

Malingering means faking. There are some people who fake pain, or at least purposely exaggerate it. This is fraud. There are schemes to defraud insurance companies—staged accidents, fraudulent patients, fraudulent chiropractors and doctors, and devious attorneys. These schemes have cost insurance companies large amounts of money. Ultimately, all consumers pay with higher premiums, and honest accident victims pay because of the distrust and suspicions that everyone is faking.

If a person with neck pain does not get better quickly and there is a lawsuit, it is too easy to attribute the poor outcome to the potential money to be gained from the suit. However, it is important to look at the scientific evidence.

Do Lawsuits Influence Outcome in Whiplash?

Many doctors and attorneys believe that personal injury litigation is at least partly responsible for the prolonged pain and suffering of patients with neck pain after a motor vehicle accident. They believe that without lawsuits and the potential for monetary reward, most patients would recover quickly and completely. The problem is sometimes even called "litigation neurosis," and there have been medical articles with titles such as "Cured by Verdict." However, as I have discussed previously, the scientific evidence shows that personal injury lawsuits do not perpetuate neck pain.

When considering such an emotional topic, it is sometimes hard to be logical. Fortunately, there is scientific research to guide us. In 1961, an article that suggested patients could be "cured by verdict" was published. This article has been used by defense lawyers and doctors to support the view that most people with neck pain and whiplash suffer from secondary gain rather than structural injury. However, the scientific evidence reaches a far different conclusion. Since 1980, at least thirty-five published studies have addressed the outcome for whiplash injuries. The overwhelming consensus is that about 15 percent to 40 percent of people with whiplash will have persistent problems. Most will have mild or moderate pain, but as many as 10 percent will have significant pain. There is scant evidence that the presence of litigation changes the outcome, nor is there evidence that settling the case improves the pain.

Some of the confusion may be due to the failure to distinguish between personal injury and workers' compensation litigation.

Personal injury litigation is legal action that results from an injury allegedly caused by someone's negligence. Common examples include car accidents and falls in supermarkets. If it can be clearly demonstrated that negligence has led to the injury, these cases may be closed with single payments of money by settlement, arbitration, or trial.

Workers' compensation litigation is different, and laws vary greatly from state to state, so there is much more variability in the way these cases proceed. The workers' compensation system began with the best of intentions as "no-fault" insurance, providing coverage if a worker was injured on the job, no matter who was at fault. Employers carry workers' compensation insurance that pays for necessary medical care, provides disability payments while the injured worker is recovering, and pays for any resulting long-term disability. The employee cannot sue for anything except medical care and permanent disability, if any.

Despite the good intentions, however, the system got out of hand. The insurers' profit is based on premium payments received (and investment interest on this money), minus any money paid out, and so they need to control medical and disability costs. The injured worker needs to prove there is ongoing disability to collect weekly payments or a final settlement, and an ongoing problem to get medical care for the injury. Once again, the two sides may become adversarial. Each injured worker becomes the center of a "mini-industry" that revolves around and depends upon his or her injury. As opposed to personal injury litigation, most scientific studies have shown that workers' compensation patients do not respond to treatment as well as people with private insurance and take longer to reach maximum medical improvement.

There have been many studies that have addressed the question, "Does litigation prolong pain and/or disability for whiplash?" One study often quoted to support the idea that personal injury litigation prolongs pain and disability was published in 1956 by Dr. Nicholas Gotten, a neurosurgeon. One of Dr. Gotten's medical students tried to contact 219 patients that Dr. Gotten and his colleagues had seen in their practices over several years. The student was only able to find 100 of the 219 patients, a fact which in and of itself prevents any meaningful conclusions. The student found that only 54 of the 100 patients were pain-free. However, because about 88 percent were at least slightly better, and all had settled their legal cases, Dr. Gotten assumed that the reason they were better was because they had settled! He felt this was proof that the lawsuit was the cause of the pain. Obviously, this conclusion is not justified by their own data since almost all of their patients still had pain many years later, long after the suits were settled, and some remained significantly disabled.

In a recent study from Canada, Dr. Leora Swartzman and her associates compared two groups of whiplash patients. One group was comprised of patients who still had a lawsuit pending and the other group of patients who had all settled their cases. They found that the patients who were still involved in lawsuits had more pain than those who had settled their lawsuits. However, the researchers found no differences in the levels of disability or psychological distress between the two groups. One might be tempted to explain these facts by concluding that the still-active lawsuit increased the pain. But an equally valid explanation is that the patients had not yet settled their cases because they were more severely injured and had more pain. It is also important to know that patients who had settled still had significant pain and impairment, although it was less than those who had not settled.

There are some good studies from England, where most patients are in the national health care system and are easy to follow for long periods. In 1983, Dr. Norris, of Northern General Hospital, Sheffield, England and Dr. Watt, of British Royal Infirmary, Bristol, England, reviewed the results of sixty-one patients followed for whiplash injuries. There were forty-one who had personal injury lawsuits. They found no change in the patients' symptoms after the claims were settled. Two other doctors reevaluated the same patients eight to twelve years later and found that, long after litigation had been settled, only 12 percent had completely recovered, and 48 percent still had pain that interfered with normal activities.

In a 1993 British study, Drs. Parinar and Raymakers published a report about patients they had seen previously for legal opinions, but not for treatment. They invited 204 people to return for reevaluation eight years after the initial consultation and 100 came in. Based on their data, they, too, concluded that lawsuits did not influence the timing or degree of recovery. The fact that only half were reevaluated does diminish the quality of the work, however.

Several years ago, we conducted our own research to learn more about the possible effects of lawsuits on recovery from whiplash syndrome. We carefully analyzed a group of patients with whiplash who were referred for treatment by their attorneys because they were not getting better. There were eleven patients with only neck pain and twenty-three patients with both neck and low back pain; all injuries stemmed from motor vehicle accidents. We analyzed pain and function by using specialized questionnaires. The patients were treated with the same aggressive conservative care program described elsewhere in this book, which included strengthening exercises, body mechanics training, medications, spinal injections, and occasionally psychotherapy. None of the patients required surgery, and most of the patients did well. We saw significant improvements in both pain and function. In fact, nearly all patients returned to normal function. Although most patients still had mild pain at the end of treatment, it was not enough to interfere with their daily lives. These very favorable results were obtained even though none of the lawsuits had been settled.

Some excellent researchers, however, feel the role of litigation might be quite important. In a study published in *The New England Journal Of Medicine* in April 2000, Canadian researchers studied the effects of changing from a litigation to a no-fault insurance system that does not include payments for pain and suffering. They did not look at individual patients, only insurance statistics. They found a small but significant decrease (28 percent) in the number of whiplash claims and a shorter period of time until the cases were settled with the no-fault system. Interestingly, these researchers also found that patients with more pain, more depression, and more impairment continue to do poorly under the no-fault insurance system. This study reminds us that with a complex problem such as whiplash, simple answers are rare, and pain, impairment, and recovery may involve structural, psychological, social, legal, and economic factors.

6
Neck-Related Headaches

Headaches are one of the most common problems in modern society, and in the computer era, they seem to have increased in frequency. In fact, many adults in the United States have at least one bad headache every month. For most people, headaches get better with rest and over-the-counter medications, but, in others, headaches occur so frequently or are so severe that they interfere with the usual activities of daily life.

Some people with recurrent headaches may fear that the pain signals the presence of cancer, stroke, or some other life-threatening condition, but it is rare for headaches to be caused by serious medical illnesses. However, people who have headaches that are very severe; that are getting progressively worse; or that are associated with fever, weight loss, fainting, confusion, or dizziness should be thoroughly evaluated by a medical doctor.

There are several types of troublesome headaches, but the three most common are migraine headache, tension-type headache, and the main focus of this chapter, neck-related (cervicogenic) headache (see table 3). The different types of headache have some symptoms in common, but because the treatment for each type may be different, it is important to try to differentiate among them.

Table 3

Characteristics of Different Types of Common Headache

	Migraine	*Tension-Type*	*Neck-Related*
Severity	Mild to severe	Mild to moderate	Mild to moderate Occasionally severe
Location	Usually one-sided	Usually both-sided	Usually one-sided
Family history	Present	Absent	Absent
Other symptoms			
Nausea	Common	Common	Occasional
Vomiting	Common	No	No
Aura	Occasional	No	No

MIGRAINE HEADACHE

A migraine is more than just a bad headache. Migraine is a specific type of headache that occurs in 10 percent to 20 percent of the population. The pain of migraine can range from mild to severe. The tendency to get migraines may be inherited, which means a migraine sufferer is likely to have a parent with migraines. Migraines are twice as common in women as in men. The frequency of headaches varies from one or two migraines a year to several per week. Headache specialists think that migraine is due to a problem with the biochemical serotonin. Abnormal levels of serotonin create changes in the brain and blood vessels that lead to the migraine headache.

Migraine pain tends to occur on one side of the head only (unilateral). The pain is constant, and often described as throbbing. Nausea and vomiting often accompany the headache. Other symptoms include weakness in an arm, generalized weakness or fatigue, partial loss of vision, strange smells, diarrhea, and difficulty speaking.

Types of Migraine

Physicians classify migraine into two main types. The first, migraine with aura, used to be called classic migraine. The aura is a warning symptom that begins before the headache, and then fades when the head pain starts. There are several types of auras. With visual auras, the person sees spots, flickering lights, or funny shapes. Other people may experience strange smells, weakness in an arm or leg, dizziness, or numbness. The second type is migraine without aura, formerly called common migraine. It is the more common type of migraine, and obviously is not associated with aura. In both migraine with aura and migraine without aura, the patterns of pain are similar.

Treatment of Migraine

The goals of the management of migraine are to decrease the frequency and severity of headaches (preventive treatment) and to relieve a headache that has already begun (symptomatic treatment). Most patients need both types of treatment.

PREVENTIVE TREATMENT

One important preventive measure is the avoidance of known triggers of migraine. Some people have no known triggers, but exposure to triggers will set off migraine in susceptible persons. Different people have different triggers, but some of the possible triggers of migraine are psychological stress, exposure to cigarette smoke, certain foods, and birth control pills. In addition to avoiding obvious migraine triggers, stress reduction techniques, biofeedback, and restful, restorative sleep can help decrease the frequency of attacks.

Medications that decrease the frequency of headaches are called preventive or prophylactic medications (table 4). The most useful category of preventive medications are called beta-blockers, and the drug used most is nadolol. If beta-blockers do not work or if they produce too many side effects, other medications can be effective.

Table 4

Drugs Used for Prevention of Migraine Attacks

Category	Drug Names
Beta-blockers	Nadolol Propranolol
Calcium channel blockers	Verapamil
Antidepressant	Nortriptyline Amitriptyline
Ergots	Methysergide
Nonsteroidal anti-inflammatory drugs	Numerous
Anticonvulsants	Valproate Phenytoin Clonazepam

SYMPTOMATIC TREATMENT

Some people respond to simple symptomatic treatments, such as lying in a dark room, putting an ice bag on the part of the head that hurts, or using over-the-counter pain medications. Not every medication works for every patient, so the doctor and patient must work together to find the best medications. The choice of medications is determined by headache severity, frequency, duration, and effect on a person's daily life. The worse the problem, the more aggressive the treatment. When prescribing medication, the doctor will take into consideration other medical conditions the patient has. That is because some migraine medications may make other medical problems— heart disease, high blood pressure, severe diabetes, history of a stroke—worse, or cause dangerous interactions with other medications.

Medications taken to stop a headache that has already begun are called symptomatic or abortive medications. One of the major breakthroughs in the symptomatic treatment of migraine is a new class of drugs called triptans, which work by adjusting one of the biochemical abnormalities that can cause migraine. There are now several triptan drugs available as pills, nasal spray, or injection.

Nonsteroidal anti-inflammatory drugs, NSAIDs (see chapter 10), can be very effective for mild or moderate headache. If NSAIDs do not work, an oral nasal spray or injectable triptan is usually tried next. Other drugs for symptomatic treatment include Midrin, ergotamines, or, rarely, sedatives. In addition, some people may need stronger pain relievers. Paradoxically, overuse or even daily use of symptomatic medications poses the very real danger of increasing the frequency of migraines.

TENSION-TYPE HEADACHE

Almost everyone has had a headache. In fact, many of us may even accept headaches as an unavoidable part of our busy lives. The most common type of headache is called tension-type headache, and affects one in three people. When headaches occur at the end of a busy workday, they may be attributed to stress and muscle tension. The pain of tension-type headache is usually mild or moderate, and usually located on both sides of the head (bilateral). People with tension-type headaches usually describe feeling a pressing or tight sensation, but less often the pain can be throbbing, like a migraine. Nausea can occur with severe tension-type headaches, but auras or other neurological symptoms are not a part of tension-type headache. If you have tension-type headaches that are mild and infrequent, they do not usually pose a significant problem. But if the pain is severe or frequent, and interferes with the activities of daily life, then more intense treatment may be required.

For years, doctors and headache sufferers alike assumed that tension-type headaches were brought on by tense muscles in the neck and at the base of the skull, and that psychological stress caused the tension. We now know that the causes of tension-type headaches are much more complicated than simple muscle tension and stress. Investigators have found biochemical changes in the brain similar to those seen in migraine. Other evidence suggests that the pain may come from the brain itself, that any muscle pain is secondary, and that tension-type headache may actually be a form of migraine.

Patients with all three types of headaches often have tight, tender, and painful muscles. These muscle changes only add to the pain that originates in deeper brain or spinal structures.

Treatment of Tension-Type Headaches

To treat tension-type headaches, the first step is to eliminate any factors that either cause headaches or make them worse, such as bad posture, bad body mechanics, or weak neck muscles. However, this preventive care requires the same long-term commitment as the treatment of neck pain (see chapters 8 and 9). Sometimes, simple techniques such as using ice or NSAIDs will be sufficient to treat an established headache.

When these simple measures are not effective, more aggressive neck muscle strengthening and treatment with prescription medications may be necessary. The most useful medications are many of the same medications used for preventive treatment of migraine, and include the antidepressants nortriptyline and amitryptiline, as well as beta-blockers.

Although psychological stress is not the cause of tension-type headaches, it certainly can make pain worse. Therefore, stress reduction techniques (see chapter 17) and psychotherapy are often helpful. Chiropractic care and massage can also help, especially for periodic flares of head pain.

NECK-RELATED HEADACHE

Headaches due to problems in the neck are termed neck-related or cervicogenic headaches. The joints, discs, muscles, and ligaments of the neck all contain nerve endings, and when any of these structures in the upper part of the neck are injured or strained, headaches can result. The pain of neck-related headaches is usually worse at the base of the skull, and may spread to the forehead, temples, eyes, or face. Moving your neck or holding your head and neck in one position for long periods can bring on the pain or make it worse. Your neck muscles may be stiff or tender, and if this is a long-standing condition, there may be abnormal findings on neck X-rays.

Other symptoms that may accompany the pain of cervicogenic headache include nausea, vomiting, sensitivity to noise or bright lights, dizziness, blurred vision, or difficulty swallowing. Because these same symptoms can also be part of migraine, it is sometimes difficult to be sure of the headache type. Some patients who have been diagnosed with tension-type headache or migraine may have neck-related headaches, and respond to treatment of the neck; probably some who have been diagnosed with neck-related headaches have migraine.

Three recent research studies have looked at the frequency of neck-related headaches. A 1995 study from Denmark showed that neck-related headache was the diagnosis in at least 18 percent of people with more than four headaches per month and 2.5 percent of the population as a whole. A 1990 study found that neck-related headache was the diagnosis in 14 percent of people with frequent headaches. A 1993 study found neck-related headache was the diagnosis in 16 percent of people with chronic headaches. In summary, 14 percent to 18 percent of chronic headache sufferers, and 2.5 percent of the population, have neck-related headaches—literally millions of people!

Causes of Neck-Related Headaches

Several structures in the neck can cause neck-related headaches (see chapter 2). The most common causes are injuries to the discs or facet joints of the upper and middle neck. Although muscle spasm may add to the overall pain, it is rarely the primary problem.

DISC INJURY

Discs are not just shock absorbers. Their more important function is to provide much of the stability for the vertebrae above and below them. The outer layer of the disc is the anulus, which has a very rich nerve supply that can be stimulated if the anulus develops tears or cracks. The anulus can be injured by a single trauma, such as a motor vehicle accident, or by chronic strain due to poor posture. Tears in the anulus can cause inflammation, which further stimulates the nerves in the anulus. Soon, even the weight of the head puts more pressure on the weakened anulus than it can support, stimulates the nerves in the wall of the anulus, and causes more pain.

Most neck-related headaches due to disc injury usually come from the upper two segments (C2/3, C3/4) of the neck. Occasionally, discs in the middle of the neck can cause headache.

FACET JOINTS

The facet joints can also be a cause of troublesome headaches, because they are so easily injured. Facet joints look, act, and sometimes even sound like knuckles. When the facet joints begin to wear, they may pop or crack—noises that are not dangerous.

Normally, the facet joints bear a smaller portion of the weight of the head than the discs. The joints contain cartilage, a joint lining, and a rich supply of nerve endings, just like other joints of the body. And, like other joints, they can wear down, become inflamed, and start hurting. The diagnosis is confirmed by numbing the nerves that go to the joint. If the pain is relieved temporarily, it is probable that the joint is the source of the pain. If so, the pain can often be helped for six to eighteen months by applying heat to the nerve, a process called radiofrequency neurotomy.

ATLANTO-OCCIPITAL AND ATLANTO-AXIAL JOINTS

At the top of the neck, where the skull and neck meet, is a joint called the atlanto-occipital joint, or the A-O joint for short. The next joint down is called the atlanto-axial joint (A-A for short). Neither of these joints has discs or facets, and either can become inflamed and cause pain. Both joints are susceptible to injury in whiplash. Chronic pain from the A-O or A-A joints may respond well to improvements in posture and good body mechanics. Chiropractic may be helpful. Cortisone injections are not as successful for this area of the spine, and neurotomy cannot be performed in this region.

MUSCLE AND LIGAMENT INJURY

About two-thirds of people with recurring headaches complain of muscle stiffness, or spasms, but that does not mean the muscles are the main cause of pain. For example, pressing on the neck muscles and causing pain also puts pressure on the facet joints, which lie just below the muscle, and so it is not possible to identify the origin of the tenderness.

There is no doubt that injuries to muscles and ligaments can cause head pain, but muscle and ligament injuries usually heal in one to three weeks. If you have ever had a "pulled muscle," you know that after a few weeks, the pain is better. It is rare for muscle or ligament pain to be chronic, severe, or disabling. The muscles of the head and neck are no different—acute muscle strains heal quickly.

However, an injury to a disc or facet joint can cause overlying muscles to go into spasm as a reaction to the deeper injury, adding to the overall pain. Discs and facet joints are far more vulnerable to injury and far more likely to cause chronic pain than muscles and ligaments. Good scientific studies have proven joints and discs can cause chronic neck pain, but there are none to show that the neck muscles or liaments can.

GREATER OCCIPITAL NEURALGIA

The greater occipital nerve, situated at the base of the skull, runs through a muscle called the splenius capitis. In many patients with neck-related headaches, this muscle is tender, and the nerve may be irritated. If a local anesthetic is injected into the muscle and around the nerve, the headache may improve. This has led many doctors to conclude that the nerve is the source of the pain, and that the nerve is being squeezed by the tight muscle. On occasion, doctors perform surgery to relieve the pressure on the nerve, but the results are not very predictable.

Treatment of Neck-Related Headaches

There is no single best treatment of neck-related headaches. There is, of course, nothing better than prevention. Paying attention to those postures or activities that seem to precipitate headaches, and then changing or avoiding them, is an important first step. Once a headache is established, however, there are many things you can do, ranging from specific postures to relieve pressure on your neck, neck first aid, to medications. Neck first aid (see chapter 7) can be very useful for neck-related headaches.

POSTURE

Proper alignment of the head and neck minimizes the forces on the discs, facet joints, and other structures. Using bad posture, especially when sitting for prolonged periods, is one of the most common causes of neck-related headaches. Improving posture often improves pain.

Good neck posture starts with good low back posture (see chapter 9). It is important to sit up straight, allowing your lower back to keep its normal curve, thus balancing the rest of the spine. Your chest should be up, with your shoulders retracted slightly, and your chin parallel to the floor. Forward bending should occur mostly at an imaginary hinge at the base of the skull, not the lower neck.

STRENGTHENING

If the head and neck are perfectly aligned and balanced, there would be no need for the muscles and ligaments to do any work. But it is nearly impossible to be in perfect position all of the time, and so the muscles and ligaments must partially support the head and neck. Strong muscles are able to hold the head and neck in proper position; weak muscles cannot. Poor posture places strain on the discs and joints and causes pain. Strong muscles are essential to good posture, and a program for strengthening the muscles is detailed in chapter 8.

MEDICATIONS

If pain gets bad enough, most people will try medications. The most useful over-the-counter medications for neck-related headaches are acetaminophen, ibuprofen, and naproxen. However, there are much stronger medications that can be helpful, but they require a doctor's prescription (see chapter 10).

INJECTIONS

There are several types of injections that can be helpful for neck-related headaches (see chapter 3). There are two major categories of therapeutic injections—steroid injections and injections that heat or freeze a nerve (neurotomy) to stop it from conducting pain.

SURGERY

Surgery should be the last thing to consider for treating neck-related headaches, but it can be helpful in patients with severe pain who have not responded to nonsurgical treatments. To decide if surgery might help and to plan the correct surgery, the exact source of the pain must be located, which requires sophisticated testing with X-rays, MRI scans, facet joint injections, and discography (see chapter 3).

Our surgeons at the SpineCare Medical Group have had encouraging results for neck-related headaches that are due to bad discs at the upper neck levels. We have found that removing the offending discs, and then fusing (joining) the adjacent vertebrae together, will relieve the pain in carefully selected patients.

7

Treatment of Acute Neck Pain: Neck First Aid

Every person with chronic neck pain will have periods when pain is worse, and for some people, the fear that pain will get worse becomes a major barrier to leading a normal life. However, people who take the time to develop the resources and knowledge to treat flares can develop the confidence to live normally again. An action plan that is ready to be implemented when a flare occurs gives you back some control over your pain. If you plan in advance for flares, you'll be able to act promptly to decrease their severity and duration. I call the treatment for acute flares "neck first aid." In almost everyone, flares abate, and pain returns to baseline in a few days with the use of neck first aid.

There are four components to neck first aid: posture, analgesics, ice, and neutralization exercises, which can be remembered by the acronym P-A-I-N.

P = Posture
A = Analgesics
I = Ice
N = Neutralization

During a flare, it is a good time to reflect on what may have caused it because you may learn things that will help prevent future episodes. Virtually all activities of daily living can be done properly without precipitating a flare, but it is not always easy to make the necessary changes. Often, using proper body mechanics requires breaking a lifetime of bad habits. Remember, though, it is not *what* you do, it is *how* you do it. Virtually every activity can be done with good body mechanics, and without pain.

Contrary to popular belief, neck pain is not caused by cold drafts or changes in barometric pressure. It is caused by mechanical disturbances of your neck alignment, such as sudden awkward moves or sustained poor posture. The precipitating incident may have occurred one or two days prior to the onset of pain, and may have been very subtle.

Some of the more common examples are sitting at a computer, studying while leaning over a desk, reading in an easy chair that has no head support, sitting at a conference taking notes all day, or lying in bed with your head supported on pillows, watching television or reading. In all these positions, the head and neck are bent forward, which places strain on the discs and perhaps the facet joints.

Activities that may be more likely to strain the joints or ligaments in the rear of the neck are those that require sustained or repetitive overhead work. Examples include loading or unloading overhead shelves, changing lightbulbs, and painting the ceiling.

POSTURE

Neck posture is the position of your head and neck in relation to each other and in relation to your chest and upper back. In chapter 9, I discuss proper neck and head posture in detail. In this section, I present neck–first aid postures and positions. Good posture is essential for the prevention and treatment of neck pain, but it is even more important during flares.

Neck Rest Position

The "neck rest position" was described by Dr. David Fardon, a spine specialist, in his 1983 book *Free Yourself from Neck Pain and Headache*. In the neck rest position, your neck bears little or no weight, which minimizes the stresses on your discs and joints and relieves the pain of a flare. The neck rest position should be used for about fifteen minutes every two hours or so during flares, and may require breaks during work or other activities. The neck rest position is also useful as a preventive measure during periods of prolonged sitting or other sustained postures that may strain the neck.

To get into the neck rest position, lie on your back facing up on a firm surface such as a carpeted floor (figure 11). Bend your hips and knees, but keep your feet flat on the floor, parallel to each other. Place a tightly rolled dish towel under your neck near the base of your skull. Let the muscles of your neck, shoulders, and upper back relax. Then close your eyes, take a slow, deep breath, hold it for a few seconds, and then let the air out slowly. With each breath, let the tension flow out of your muscles. Stay in the neck rest position for fifteen minutes before returning to normal activities.

Neutral Sitting Posture

The discs, joints, muscles, and ligaments of the neck are under the least amount of strain when the neck is balanced in a neutral position (see chapter 9). Your low back posture must be correct to allow the rest of the spine to be properly positioned

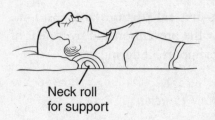

Neck roll
for support

Figure II
Neck rest position. A rolled
towel is placed under the neck
for support. The neck rest
position unloads the discs,
joints, and muscles of the
neck, and is a good position
for relaxing, sleeping, and
pain control ("neck first aid").

to achieve the low back position that forms the best base for
the rest of your spine. Envision your lower back as a C-shaped
curve with the closed side of the C facing the belly button and
the open side of the C facing backward.

Sit in a good chair with good lumbar posture. Gently pull
back your shoulders and shoulder blades and bring your chest
up, which will bring your neck up to the correct position. Keep
your chin parallel to the floor. The combined effect of good
lumbar curve, holding your chest up with shoulders slightly
back and your chin slightly retracted and parallel to the floor, is
the neutral spine position. It should feel natural and not
strained. Neck motion should occur at a pivot point or hinge at
the very top of the neck at the base of the skull, not in the middle of the neck. When you read, keep the book or reading
materials at eye level. Do not read in bed unless your head is
fully supported and you are able to hold your reading material
straight in front of you at eye level. There are more details
about reading and working at a desk in chapter 9. Check yourself every few minutes to be sure you have not slumped down,
and correct to the neutral position if you have. Avoid extending
your neck to look up overhead. Look straight ahead. If you
have to reach over your head, get up first, and, if necessary,
stand on a secure stool or ladder and bring your body (and
therefore your eyes) up to the work surface.

ANALGESICS (PAIN MEDICATIONS)

Pain medications are discussed in detail in chapter 10, but it is worthwhile to mention a few points about the use of medications for acute flares as a part of neck first aid. The over-the-counter analgesics, ibuprofen (Advil), naproxen (Aleve), and acetaminophen (Tylenol), can provide good pain relief, especially when used in conjunction with the other elements of neck first aid.

Medications should be taken at moderately high doses and on a regular schedule. The interval between doses depends on the drug. Ibuprofen and acetaminophen work best when taken every six hours, and naproxen can be taken every eight to twelve hours. Taking medications "by the clock," rather than when waiting until the pain worsens, is more effective because then you are maintaining a more constant level of the medication in your system. I recommend continuing the medication for two or three days after the pain has subsided to keep the inflammation down.

ICE

Ice is very helpful for pain control, and its value is often underappreciated. Ice can relieve pain, decrease inflammation, and is available everywhere. Ordinary ice cubes in a freezer bag work well, so there is no need for special ice bags or prepackaged "blue ice." Regular ice is also safer, since it is far less likely to "ice burn" the skin. Put several ice cubes in a freezer bag, then wrap the bag in a thin dish towel and place it directly over the painful area for about fifteen minutes. You can repeat ice treatment every three to four hours. Although ice may feel uncomfortable when you first put the pack on your skin, the cold will soon penetrate into painful and inflamed tissues and ease pain for several hours. You can pack empty freezer bags for ice treatment when traveling.

Another effective technique is ice massage, but you'll have to prepare in advance by freezing water in a Styrofoam cup. To use it, peel back the edges of the cup, which provides a large ice cube in a holder. Then rub the ice back and forth over the painful area until the ice is melted. Obviously, this is messier than a bag of ice, but it works better for some people.

"NEUTRALIZATION" EXERCISES

Exercises to treat acute neck pain differ from the strengthening exercises that are a major component of the long-term treatment program. These exercises for flares are modified from those presented in the 1983 book *Treat Your Own Neck*, by Robin McKenzie. McKenzie, a world-renowned physical therapist, recommends five exercises, performed in the order listed: chin retractions, neck extensions, neck flexions, side bending, and neck rotations.

I have termed the exercises for acute pain "neutralization" exercises, because the goal is to neutralize the effects of the bad neck position(s) that caused the pain. You neutralize the pain by exercising your neck in the direction opposite to the one that caused the pain. For example, if your flare was caused by sitting or lying with your head and neck bent forward in flexion, then extension exercises are most likely to neutralize the pain. Conversely, if the flare was caused by painting the ceiling or changing lightbulbs with your head and neck in extension, then flexion exercises are most likely to help.

In my experience, the most valuable exercises are chin retractions, neck extensions, and neck flexions. These exercises can be done sitting or lying down. In general, if you have slight to moderate pain, you should do the exercises seated. If your pain is severe or does not respond to the exercises done seated, do the exercises lying down.

When you are in pain, exercising is probably the last thing you want to do. Chances are, you would rather lie around, take some pills, and be left alone. But remember that "discipline takes discipline." If you try the neutralization exercises and they work, in the future you will be more likely to begin them at the first sign of increased pain. In fact, it is easier to bring the acute flare under control if the exercises are begun at the first symptoms of worsening pain, because the longer the pain is present, the longer it will take to get better.

Neutralization exercises may initially cause an increase in pain in some people. As you do each exercise, you should gradually increase the end point of the range of motion, beginning at a position that causes just a slight increase in pain. That is the limit of the range for you at that time. After a few sets of exercises, your pain should begin to decrease and your range of motion should increase. If the pain is getting worse, then either you have chosen the wrong exercise, there is an error in your technique, or the problem is not responsive to exercise. If you are having pain in the arm when you begin to exercise, the pain should start receding toward your neck or midline, which is called centralization, and is a good sign. If the pain spreads outward toward the arm, this is not a good sign, and it may be time to seek medical help.

Which Neutralization Exercises Are Best?

When choosing exercises for your acute neck pain, remember that they must be individualized for your particular situation. Once again, it is important to emphasize exercises that work the neck in the direction opposite to the position that caused the pain. When pain is caused by flexion positions (head down), extension exercises should work better. When pain is caused by extension postures (head up and back), then flexion exercises usually work better. Flexion exercises stress the backs of the discs and ease pressure on the facet joints, while extension exercises increase the load on the facets and nerve canals, but ease the load on the backs of discs. Some people have both problems, and need both types of exercise directions. It takes some trial and error to decide which exercises are best. *do seated*

Chin retractions are one of the most important exercises for all patients, and are the first exercise to do. They are followed by either neck extensions (most often) or neck flexions (less often). Finally, rotations feel good for many patients, and are appropriate unless they make the pain worse. I have seen mixed results with the lateral extension exercises and rarely emphasize them.

When you do many of these exercises, you may hear popping noises or feel cracking sensations, which probably are due to gas being expelled from the joints. This is not dangerous, and, like cracking your knuckles, will do no harm.

Neutral Sitting Posture

Most of the neutralization exercises are done in the neutral sitting posture or position (see chapter 9).

1. Sit in a firm chair with good low back support.
2. Curve your low back inward toward your belly button.
3. Lift up your chest.
4. Pull back your shoulders gently.
5. Keep your chin parallel to the floor.

Chin Retractions

Chin retractions can be helpful for pain that arises from discs, joints, or soft tissues. Physical therapists sometimes call this exercise "dorsal glides." During an acute flare, it is a good idea to repeat chin retractions every two to three hours. It is also a good preventive exercise for long-term maintenance.

Chin Retractions (figure 12)

1. Starting posture: neutral sitting posture.
2. Exercise:

    Slowly but steadily retract your chin as far back as it will go comfortably.

    Keep your chin parallel to the floor; do not tilt your head backward.

    Keep your chin back and slowly count to five.
3. Relax.
4. Repeat the chin retractions five times.

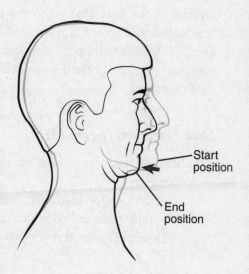

Figure 12

Pain neutralization exercise. Chin retractions. While sitting with good posture, retract your chin gently backward but kept parallel to the floor. This exercise is repeated five times, and during flares should be repeated many times during the day.

Start position

End position

It is sometimes even more helpful to repeat the chin retractions, but increase the amount of retraction by gently pushing your chin back using your hands.

If doing chin retractions while sitting causes you to have more pain, do them lying down in the neck rest position. Before starting, check to make sure that your chin is perpendicular to the floor. Retract your chin (and head) backward toward the floor or mattress as far back as you can. Hold the position for a slow count to five, and then relax. Perform ten repetitions. Do chin retractions every two to three hours during the day. When your pain begins to decrease, change to the seated position for doing the exercise.

Neck Extensions

Neck extensions are performed following chin retractions. People who have had angina, heart attack, or a stroke should not do this exercise until they have discussed it with their doctors, because extension of the neck may put pressure on arteries in the neck that go to the brain. This is not a problem unless the artery is narrowed by arteriosclerosis. However, if you experience significant dizziness during the exercise, stop and consult a physician before resuming extension exercises.

Neck Extensions (figure 13)

1. Starting position: neutral sitting posture.
2. Exercise:
   > After a set of chin retractions, hold your chin in the fully retracted position.
   > Slowly lift your chin up toward the ceiling.

Let your neck and head extend back as far as they can
go comfortably.

When you are in your fully extended neck position,
gently rotate your head one to two inches to the
right and then to the left. Rotate six times in each
direction while pulling your neck slightly farther
backward into more extension and increasing the
amount of rotation.

3. After ten seconds, return to the neutral position.

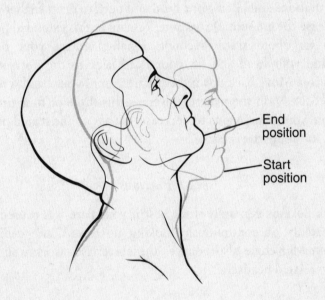

End
position

Start
position

Figure 13

Pain neutralization exercise. Neck extensions. While sitting with good
posture, and after doing chin retractions, bend your head backward
and then rotate side to side. This exercise is particularly useful for neck
pain brought on by prolonged reading or working at a computer.

4. Relax.

5. Do the exercise ten times to complete the set.

If you are in too much pain to do this exercise sitting, you can do it lying on a bed. Move your body up to the edge of the mattress until the tops of your shoulders are just off the end of the mattress. Place one hand behind your head for support, and gently lower your head backward off the end of the mattress as far as you can. Remove your hand. Rotate your head about one inch to the left and then to the right. Repeat six gentle rotations and allow your head and neck to drop farther and increase the amount of rotation. Remain in this extended position for about thirty seconds. Finally, replace your hand behind your head and lift your head back to the horizontal position. Move back down the mattress until your head is resting securely on the mattress. Repeat this three or four times. When your pain begins to decrease, change to the seated position for doing the exercise.

Neck Flexions

Neck flexions generally work best if your flare was caused by repeatedly or continuously looking up toward the ceiling. Robin McKenzie also believes these exercises work well for neck-related headaches.

Neck Flexions (figure 14)

1. Starting position: neutral sitting posture.
2. Exercise:
    Perform a set of chin retractions.
    Gently and slowly allow your head to drop forward toward your chest.

Keep your chin retracted.

Place both hands with the fingers interlocked behind your head with your elbows pointed toward the ground. Do not pull actively, but instead allow gravity to pull on your hands and arms, which will bring your chin closer to the breastbone. You may feel pulling in the lower part of the back of the neck.

3. Remain in the full flexion position for about ten seconds and then return to the neutral position.

4. Relax.

Figure 14

Pain neutralization exercise. Neck flexions. While sitting with good posture, and after doing chin retractions, bend your head gently forward so your chin touches your breastbone.

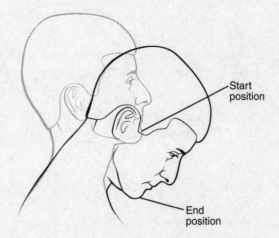

Start position

End position

Neck Rotations

The theory behind performing neck rotations is to increase the range of motion and decrease pain. If you get some pain relief with neck rotations, then it is fine to add them to your exercise program.

5. Do the exercise ten times to complete the set.
6. Repeat one set of chin retractions.
7. Repeat one set of neck extensions.

Neck Rotations (figure 15)

1. Starting position: neutral sitting posture.
2. Exercise:
   Do a set of chin retractions.
   Keep your chin parallel to the floor and retracted.

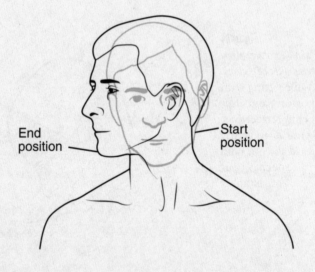

End position —   — Start position

Figure 15

Pain neutralization exercise. Neck rotations. While sitting with good posture, and with your chin retracted, rotate your head in one direction as far as you can. If it is painful, stop at a point just after the pain increases.

Rotate your chin toward your shoulder just to the point of pain.

Hold for five seconds at the maximum rotation.

3. Relax.
4. Do a set of extensions.

Side Bending

Side bending may be most useful when your neck pain is localized to one side of the neck. The goal is to be able to gradually increase your ability to bend toward the painful side.

Side Bending

1. Starting position: neutral sitting posture.
2. Exercise:

   Retract your chin.

   Slowly bend your neck sideways without turning, moving your neck closer toward the shoulder. Be sure your shoulder does not lift. Pain may increase slightly, but should not increase significantly.
3. Hold this position for ten seconds.
4. Breathe slowly and deeply while your head is at its end-range position. It is helpful to place the hand closest to the painful side (right-sided neck pain, right hand) on top of your head, and gently pull your head down. Keep the chin retracted.
5. Relax.
6. Perform ten repetitions.

When the pain has centralized into the middle of the neck primarily, then you can eliminate this exercise.

Scapulae Pinching

If you spend all day sitting, your shoulders and upper back tend to round forward, and this pushes your head and neck forward. Scapulae or shoulder blade pinching is a way to reverse slumped shoulders.

Scapulae Pinching (figure 16)

1. Starting position: neutral standing posture.
2. Exercise:
   Do a set of chin retractions.
   Let your arms dangle at your sides.

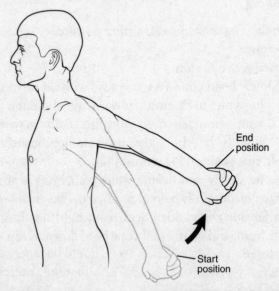

Figure 16

Pain neutralization exercise. Scapulae pinching. While sitting with good posture, interlock your hands with the palms facing each other and your elbows straight. Then raise your hands upward toward your shoulders.

Clasp your hands behind your buttocks by interlocking the fingers, palms facing each other.

Slowly raise your arms up toward your waist, keeping your elbows straight.

Hold at maximum comfortable height for five seconds.

3. Relax.
4. Repeat four or five times.

OTHER TREATMENT OPTIONS

Chiropractic Care

Chiropractic care (chapter 12) may be especially helpful for some patients with acute neck pain or acute flares of chronic neck pain. Chiropractic consists of a combination of mobilization, manipulation, and soft tissue massage. It works best for facet joint pain, soft tissue pain, and possibly for tears in the wall of a disc. If your pain is primarily in the neck or between the shoulder blades, then it is reasonable to try a chiropractor. However, if you have a significant amount of arm pain or any arm weakness, then I do not recommend chiropractic treatment, because there may be a disc herniation pressing on a nerve. In this case, evaluation by a medical doctor is important, but if there is no evidence of nerve damage on the doctor's examination, then chiropractic care is safe.

Chiropractic treatment may be needed two or three times per week for two or three weeks, and should be tapered to zero by six to eight weeks, while strengthening exercises are resumed. There is no evidence that a longer period of treatment will improve the long-term outcome, although some chiropractors recommend maintenance of the spine with regular treatments over many months to years.

Cervical Collars

Cervical collars can be useful during flares of pain, but obviously, to be able to use a collar at the onset of a flare, you must have purchased it ahead of time. All collars restrict motion to some extent, but if you are going to use a collar, choose one that works. The best collars require a physician's prescription. Soft foam collars do not adequately restrict motion, and almost all other types of collars are better. The Philadelphia collar, made of Styrofoam, is lightweight, easy to fit, easy to use, comfortable, and inexpensive. It is reasonable for short-term use. The best collar, however, is the Miami-J collar. It is easy to fit and immobilizes the neck well. Although it is not as comfortable as the lighter collars, it works much better.

Although neck collars are not good long-term treatment, they can be useful in the short-term treatment of flares, especially for the person who must continue to work or drive despite increased pain. Collars should be used in conjunction with other neck–first aid measures.

Traction

Many people with neck pain feel as if their bones and joints are rubbing against each other. Although this is not what is happening, some people feel better when the neck is pulled. Traction is any system to pull on the neck along the long axis of the vertebrae.

There are two ways to apply traction. Manual traction is performed by another person using his or her hands to pull on the patient's neck. It usually is performed by chiropractors or physical therapists, but if there is good relief, these professionals could train a patient's family member or friend to apply manual traction at home.

There are several commercial traction devices available, usually by prescription. The oldest is an over-the-door system in which a harness is placed around the head. A rope attached to the harness and a pulley goes over a door, and a counterweight is on the other side. By increasing the counterweight, you are able to apply more traction. However, there are better systems available. Pulley systems used while you lie on the floor keep the angle of the pull correct. These systems also use a harness around the head, but you apply the counterweight by using your own legs or arms to exert the force. It is much easier to judge and regulate the amount of traction you use, so the systems are much safer. There are also pneumatic systems that inflate like a blood pressure cuff to apply more traction.

If you have access to a traction device, and know that it has provided relief in the past, then this can be a part of your neck–first aid program. You should try traction first under the direct supervision of a chiropractor or physical therapist. If you experience relief, then it is worthwhile to rent a unit for home use. If the home unit works, then it may be cost-effective to purchase it.

Tender-Point Therapy

Many people with acute pain have tender points in their muscles. Although the tender muscles are not usually the underlying cause of the problem, the muscles can be painful if they are overworked, strained from being held too long in a single position, or are guarding an underlying injury to a deeper structure. The treatment of the tender muscle points can provide some pain relief while the underlying tissues heal.

Tender points in muscles can often be treated with massage and acupressure. In addition, there are small wooden tender-point treatment devices available in many health food stores.

8
Treatment of Neck Pain: Exercise and Strength Training

The treatment for neck pain is simple:

- Use good body mechanics at rest and while active.
- Strengthen your neck and upper back muscles so you can use good body mechanics.

This chapter provides the rationale for an exercise program to strengthen your muscles and the details to implement it without the need for expensive gyms or complex equipment. The exercise program can be readily incorporated into a busy lifestyle. In chapter 9, I discuss the essentials of posture and body mechanics, which go hand in hand with strength training.

There is no easy way to get strong—you have to exercise, and it takes time and commitment. Too many people feel that they cannot afford the time to exercise, but they fail to factor in the time they lose when they stay home from work or miss family or other social events because of neck pain. Each person with neck pain has the choice to exercise on a regular basis, use good body mechanics, and feel better; or find reasons to avoid exercise, stay weak, use poor body mechanics and hurt. Exercise takes discipline, and discipline takes discipline.

In my clinical experience, in the beginning of a strength-training program, it requires at least an hour per day, three or four days a week for about two months before there is a meaningful difference in strength and pain reduction. It may take even longer for people who start out very weak or who find their bad habits especially hard to break. After that, it takes only about half the time to stay in shape—far less time than the average person spends watching television or reading magazines. When progress seems slow, remember: if it were easy, it would be easy.

SEEKING HELP

Some people are not able to learn the principles of strength training and body mechanics on their own, and require professional help from a physical therapist, a chiropractor, or an exercise trainer. Other patients require more sophisticated care from a physician who specializes in spine problems for advice, medications, or spinal injections to provide temporary pain relief so they can exercise. However, no treatment offered by any health professional can succeed in the long run if the injured person is not willing to accept responsibility and devote the time and energy it takes to get better. It is your neck, stick it out!

MUSCLE STRENGTHENING: THE BASIC CONCEPTS

The goal of exercise is to develop sufficient muscle strength to be able to hold your head and neck in positions of good posture at rest and during activity. During strength training, your muscles must be worked hard enough to get stronger, but not too hard to risk injury. Good technique is important to protect the muscles, discs, and joints.

Isometric and Isotonic Exercises

Muscles can be strengthened by isometric or isotonic exercises. In isometric exercises, muscles contract against resistance, but the joints controlled by those muscles do not move. An example is pressing your palms together firmly in front of your chest, which causes contraction of the muscles in the front of your chest (pectoral muscles). Another example would be lying on the floor facing up and pushing your head down against the floor. Because you are pushing against an unmovable surface (the floor), your head and neck do not move when the muscles in the back of your neck contract. Isometric exercises improve muscle strength and tone, but do not usually increase muscle bulk.

In isotonic exercises, when the muscles contract, the joints they control move. An example is an exercise called biceps curls. You sit with a weight in one hand, bend your elbow, and then relax it. This is an isotonic exercise to strengthen the large muscle of your upper arm, the biceps.

Repetitions and Resistance

To increase your strength, you need to gradually increase the work your muscles do during exercise. With isometric exercises, you can either increase the duration of the exercise, add weights to the resistance, or exert more force when pushing against immovable resistance. With isotonic exercises, you can work harder in two ways—either by increasing the number of times the exercise is repeated (repetitions) or by increasing the weight (resistance). To increase muscle tone and endurance, you should increase repetitions or duration of the exercise. To increase power and bulk, you should increase resistance. For most people with neck pain, increased tone and endurance are probably more important than increased bulk. That said, you will probably get the most benefit if you emphasize increasing the number of repetitions and duration, but gradually increasing the resistance.

Strength training is done in sets. One set is the number of repetitions or the duration of the isometric exercise. There may be ten repetitions (reps, for short) or an isometric hold of thirty seconds per set. To complete an exercise, you may do three sets of ten repetitions each. For some workouts, the resistance may be changed between sets. There may be one set of ten easy reps, a second set of ten reps with greater resistance, and then a third easy set.

MUSCLE GROUPS

The muscles in the back of the neck are called the posterior or extensor muscles, and they are the major muscles responsible for holding your head upright and balanced. The muscles in the front of the neck are called the anterior or flexor muscles. They contribute to balancing your head and also play a significant role in the fine adjustments of position. The flexor and extensor muscles work together to achieve a delicate balance in posture and movement, and so both muscle groups must be strong.

The muscles between your shoulder blades are called the interscapular muscles, and they form the platform for your head and neck. The interscapular muscles are one of the weakest links in the neck muscle chain, possibly because they are not used much in the activities of daily living. We do most things in front of us, such as carrying groceries, books, boxes, or children, and so we constantly use the muscles of our arms and front of the chest. These same muscles are emphasized in the gym with push-ups or chest presses, but very few people do exercises to work the interscapular muscles. The chest muscles get stronger, while the extensor muscles do not change, which leads to an imbalance. The stronger chest muscles subtly pull the chest forward and round the shoulders, so the head and neck are pulled forward and out of balance. The resulting slumped posture puts strain on the structures of the neck and may lead to chronic neck pain. The treatment is to restore balance by strengthening the weaker interscapular muscles and then using the strength to improve posture and movement patterns.

EQUIPMENT

Some exercises will be performed on a carpeted floor or exercise mat. Others will be done over the side of a bed, piano bench, or a kitchen chair without arms. In order to check that you are using proper form, it can be helpful to work out in front of a large mirror. For timed exercises, you'll need a clock, wristwatch, or kitchen timer.

To provide the resistance necessary for some of the exercises, a long stocking or pantyhose filled with sand, dirt, or stones works well. As you get stronger, you can easily add more weight. For other exercises, you will need a length of rubber tubing, which can be bought at a medical supply store. They are available in different tensile or resistance strengths. It is useful to buy a wide variety so you can experiment and find which are right for you, and by using tubes of increasing resistance, you will be able to increase the intensity of the workouts over time.

EXERCISE PROGRESSION

Beginning Your Workout Program

To begin a strengthening program, you first need to select the number of repetitions, the number of sets, and the duration of time or the amount of resistance for each exercise. Although there is no perfect method to choose the starting point for each variable, one way is to determine your maximum capacity for each exercise you are going to do, and then to begin the workouts at one-half to two-thirds of this maximum. However, if your pain begins to increase significantly during the testing, stop the exercise, and consider the point where pain increased significantly to be your maximum. Workouts are begun a few days later with three sets of one-half to two-thirds of the maximum. If the test caused a flare, begin at one-half, but if it did not, begin at two-thirds.

For example, the exercise to strengthen the muscles in the front of the neck is the anterior isometric head lift (see page 130). While lying on your back, you raise your head about one-quarter inch straight up from the mat and hold the position until your muscles fatigue, which is your maximum time. The symptoms of muscle fatigue are a rubbery feeling, twitching, or cramping. Then, to begin the strength training, perform the repetitions of the exercise at one-half to two-thirds of your maximum time. If you were able to hold the position for twenty seconds, your starting time will be ten to twelve seconds. You can determine your maximum capacity for isotonic exercises by doing multiple repetitions of the exercise until you cannot do more or the muscles feel very fatigued.

For people who are very sensitive to exercise, I recommend this slightly less aggressive method. Do a set of repetitions or hold an isometric position until the muscle just *begins* to feel fatigued, or pain gets slightly worse. Then begin the workout at about 20 percent less intensity. If the fatigue begins after thirty seconds, begin the workout with three sets of about twenty-four seconds each. If fatigue begins after twenty reps, begin the workout with three sets of sixteen reps. If this proves too aggressive, rest for a week and then resume at only 50 percent to 60 percent of your former level.

Increasing Resistance and Duration

In order to get stronger, you must increase the resistance, the number of repetitions, or the duration of each exercise. However, as you no doubt already know, if you exercise muscles that are weak and deconditioned, you will usually experience a temporary increase in pain and stiffness. There may be an increase in your usual pain, or you may get new pains in your muscles or ligaments. You can treat your increased pain by using the techniques of neck first aid described in chapter 7 with posture, ice, analgesics, and neutralization exercises. In most instances, the increased pain will resolve in a day or two, and it will be time to return to exercising.

Some people are extremely sensitive to exercise, and get worse at very low levels of strength training. These highly sensitive people need professional supervision from a physical therapist who can individualize a program and carefully monitor it for subtle errors in technique, perhaps substituting alternative exercises to strengthen the same muscles.

Most people can begin with the isometric exercises described on the following pages. If you do not have a significant flare of pain, then you can increase the exercises by 10 percent each week. For the isokinetic exercises, the amount of weight should be increased by 10 percent each week. Although this may seem very slow at first, these 10 percent increases are like compound interest, and after a few weeks, you will see significant improvement in strength. At the end of each set, the muscle should feel somewhat fatigued but not exhausted, and the third set should be more difficult to complete than the first. This means that you are working at the appropriate level of difficulty.

When you are able to hold an isometric position for more than two to three minutes, it is time to add to or increase the resistance. The amount of weight to add for each exercise is discussed in the following pages.

Frequency of Training

Muscle physiologists have taught us that in order for muscles to get stronger, you must alternate hard workouts with periods of rest, and a hard workout every other day is preferable to an easy daily workout. Begin an exercise routine twice per week for two or three weeks, and then increase to three or four times per week.

SPECIFIC MUSCLE-STRENGTHENING EXERCISES

In the following sections, I explain how to perform the exercises to strengthen the various muscles. For some muscle groups, I have discussed more than one exercise. However, there is no need to do them all. Any one of the group will do. If one is too difficult or causes a flare, try the other. Start with the one that seems most comfortable for you.

Flexor Muscle Strength Training

The neck flexor muscles are located in the front (anterior) of the neck, and play a major role in the stabilizing and balancing of your head and neck. They are also important for good head and neck balance and a fine sense of positioning. These muscles are weak in almost everyone, but especially in people with neck pain.

Exercise 1. *Anterior Isometric Head Lift*

- Workout surface: Carpeted floor or mat.
- Equipment: Timer or a watch with a second hand.
- Isometric time: Begin at one-half to two-thirds of your maximum.
- Position: Lie on the floor or mat with both knees bent, both feet flat on the floor and about six inches apart, and your hands at your sides.
- Exercise: Keeping your chin perpendicular to the floor, raise your head very slightly (about one-eighth or one-quarter inch) off the floor or mat, just enough to slip a piece of ordinary cardboard between your head and the surface but not enough to slide your hand in.
  DO NOT BEND (FLEX) YOUR NECK OR HEAD.
- Hold this position for the designated time.
- Rest.
- Repeat two more times for a total of three sets.
- Progression of resistance: When this exercise becomes easy, and you can hold the position for two to three minutes, then you should add some weight. Begin by adding one pound of dirt or sand into a sock placed on your forehead. Increase to two and three pounds when you can hold each weight in the desired position for two to three minutes.

Extensor Muscle Strength Training

The neck extensor muscles are located in the back (posterior) of the neck, and play a major role in keeping your neck in proper position when you are reading, writing, or working at a computer. They also contribute to the stabilizing and balancing of your head and neck. These muscles are usually fairly strong, but not strong enough to support the head in proper position for long periods of

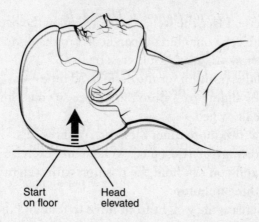

Start
on floor

Head
elevated

Figure 17

Isometric head lift to strengthen the muscles in front of your neck. While lying on the floor facing upward, lift your head about one-eighth inch from the floor, keeping your chin perpendicular to the floor.

time or under prolonged mechanical stress. The next two exercises are designed to strengthen the posterior neck muscles.

Exercise 2. Posterior Isometric Head Lift

- Workout surface: Chair without arms, piano bench, or bed.
- Equipment:
    Timer or watch with a second hand.
    Three pounds of weight, such as a stocking, sock, or freezer bag filled with three pounds of dirt or sand.
- Isometric time: Begin at one-half to two-thirds of your maximum.
- Position: Lie on the bed, chair, or bench facedown with your head, neck, and chest off the surface up to your nipple line, but keep your hips and legs on the surface.

- Exercise: Place the weight or stocking on the back of your head. Keep your chin perpendicular to the floor.
  DO NOT BEND (FLEX) YOUR NECK OR HEAD.
- Hold this position for the designated time.
- Rest by sliding back onto the surface so your chin rests on the chair or bed.
- Repeat two more times for a total of three sets.
- Progression of resistance: When this exercise becomes easy, and you can hold the position with weight for more than three minutes:

  Increase the weight from three to four and then to five pounds or

  Add chin retractions, starting with three pounds of weight on the back of the head. This converts the head lift exercise from isometric to isokinetic.

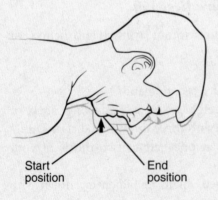

Start position   End position

Figure 18
Backward head lift to strengthen the muscles in the back of your neck. Lying facedown with your head and chest extended over the edge of a bed, retract your chin upward toward the ceiling while your chin remains perpendicular to the floor.

Exercise 3. Posterior Isometric Head Press Against the Floor

This is a simple exercise that can be done almost anywhere, even during a break at work. It is virtually the opposite of the anterior isometric head lift, and is recommended by many neck specialists. It could be hard to judge the amount of pressure to exert, which may lead to some inconsistencies in performance, but it is worth trying because it is so convenient to do.

- Workout surface: Carpeted floor or mat.
- Equipment: Sponge, washcloth, or piece of quarter-inch foam.
- Position: Lie on the floor facing up toward the ceiling. Place a folded washcloth, sponge, or foam that is about one-quarter inch thick behind your head.
- Exercise: Push down backward against the floor or carpet.
- Duration: Twenty seconds.
- Relax for thirty seconds.
- Repeat two more times for a total of three sets.

Figure 19

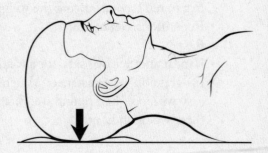

Posterior head press to strengthen the muscles in the back of your neck. While lying on the floor facing upward, with your head on a sponge or washcloth, push your head down against the floor while keeping your chin perpendicular to the floor.

Strength Training of Interscapular Muscles

The interscapular muscles are important because they form a base upon which the neck and head rest. In most people, these muscles are very weak and underdeveloped. Strong interscapular muscles complement strong neck muscles, and form the base for supporting the head.

Exercise 4. Interscapular Isotonic Strengthening Using Weights

- Workout surface: A stool about two feet high.
- Equipment: One-half, one-, and two-pound weights. (Cans of food or soup may do.)
- Position: Lie with your knees on the floor with your hips bent to 90 degrees. Place your chest on the stool. Hold your head and neck in neutral. Keep your arms dangling down toward the floor with a one-pound weight in each hand.
- Exercise: Lift your arms up perpendicular to the floor, trying to "pinch" your shoulder blades together. Hold for five to ten seconds. Bring the weights back to the floor.
- Repetitions: Set of ten.
- Rest.
- Repeat another two sets, for a total of three sets.
- Progression of resistance: When this exercise becomes easy with one-half pound weights, increase to one pound, then two pounds, etc.

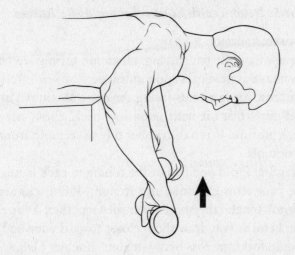

Figures 20 and 21

Interscapular strengthening for the muscles between your shoulder blades. Lying facedown over the edge of a bed and holding a one- or two-pound weight in each hand, lift both arms upward. You should feel a pinching between your shoulder blades. Figure 20 is the starting position and 21 is the end position.

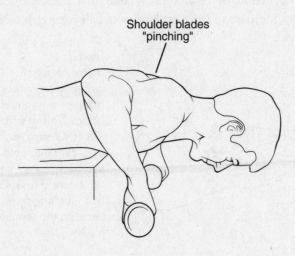

Shoulder blades "pinching"

Exercise 5. Isotonic with Elastic Tubing As Resistance

- Workout surface: A chair.
- Equipment: Elastic tubing rated for various resistances (available at medical supply stores).
- Position: Sit in a chair facing the door, about two to three feet away from it with good low back, chest, head, and neck posture. Wrap the rubber tubing securely around the doorknob.
- Exercise: Hold one end of the tubing in each hand, keeping your arms extended and straight. Pull backward, trying to "pinch" the shoulder blades together. Your elbows will bend as you draw them closer toward your body. You should feel tightness between your shoulder blades. Avoid using your arms to pull. Pull from the muscles between your shoulder blades. Keep your shoulders down! Hold for five seconds, and then slowly release.
- Repetitions: Set of ten.
- Rest.
- Repeat another two sets for a total of three sets.
- Progression of resistance: When this exercise becomes easy, increase to the next higher tensile-strength tubing.

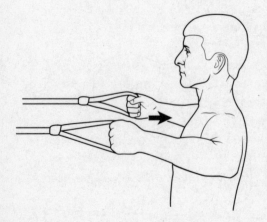

Figure 22
Seated rowing to strengthen the muscles between the shoulder blades. Sitting with elastic tubing attached to a doorknob in each hand, pull back toward your shoulders. There should be a pinching feeling between the shoulder blades.

FLEXIBILITY OR STRETCHING EXERCISES

Many doctors, chiropractors, and physical therapists emphasize flexibility in their treatment of neck pain. They often recommend flexibility exercises such as neck rotations (turning the head and neck to the left and then right), bending to the sides, and bending forward and backward. They theorize that because many patients have decreased range of motion, working to improve the range will improve the pain. Even though this might seem logical, there is no scientific evidence to support this theory. In fact, it has been shown that when strength and pain improve, range of motion improves as well without stretching exercises. Furthermore, as I have stated throughout this book, the restricted range of motion is most likely due to underlying problems with joints or discs, and efforts directed solely at improving range of motion will not provide long-term pain relief.

Some physical therapists and chiropractors feel it is important to "mobilize" stiff segments of the neck by spinal manipulative therapy (SMT). However, once again, the reason a segment feels stiff is because there is an underlying joint or disc problem. Although SMT done by an experienced practitioner poses little danger (and there is no doubt it can feel good temporarily), there will be no long-term benefits unless you also make improvements in posture and strength.

That said, flexibility exercises and stretching do feel good and can temporarily relieve some pain. The flexibility exercises I suggest are the neutralization exercises discussed in chapter 7. They provide an excellent complement to strengthening exercises, and can be done at the conclusion of the exercise routine. I recommend doing chin retractions, neck extensions with rotation, and, if it feels good, very gentle neck flexions, after each strengthening workout.

In addition, it is advantageous to develop maximum flexibility in other parts of the body. For instance, the more flexible the hamstrings and calf muscles are, the easier it is to bend correctly and thereby decrease the stresses on the neck and low back.

9

Treatment of Neck Pain: Posture and Body Mechanics

Using good body mechanics is the most important thing you can do to relieve neck pain. Body mechanics is a term used to describe the interrelationship between parts of the body during movement and at rest. With respect to the neck, body mechanics refers to the interrelationship between the head, neck, chest, upper back, and low back. As discussed in chapter 8, strength and good body mechanics go hand in hand—you must have a high level of muscle strength to use good body mechanics.

There are optimum points of balance for the head on the neck and the neck on the upper body. Proper balance of your head, neck, and upper body minimizes the stresses on the mucles, discs, and facets, so damaged tissues can heal, and pain decrease. Poor posture and body mechanics unbalance the spine, creating high stresses on the neck, and impeding healing of damaged tissues, so pain continues.

Unfortunately, our work and recreational environments are not often conducive to the use of good mechanics. We sit too long in poorly designed chairs, use desks that are too low, stare at computer monitors that are improperly placed, and ride bicycles that are poorly fitted. But thanks to the science of ergonomics, all of these factors can be changed. Ergonomics is the science devoted to the study and analysis of human work and activities of daily living, especially as they relate to the physical arrangements of our workplaces, home environments, and sports equipment. Ergonomics also can be defined as the clinical and scientific study of the use of the body in work, sports, and activities of daily living.

We have learned from the study of ergonomics that we can change our work, recreational, and home environments to maximize the opportunities to use the positions and conditions that are best for our individual bodies. This chapter outlines the basics of good posture and body mechanics to allow your neck to heal and prevent further injury.

THE LOW BACK: THE PLATFORM FOR GOOD POSTURE AND BODY MECHANICS

As you have already learned in chapter 2, the spine functions as an integrated unit, and poor posture in one part of the spine forces other parts out of alignment and balance. Your low back (lumbar spine) provides the base of support for the rest of the spine. The optimal position of the lumbar spine is a C-shaped curve, called the lumbar lordosis, that arcs inward toward the belly button. A good lumbar lordosis provides the ideal platform for the rest of the spine and also minimizes the stresses on the discs and facet joints of the low back. To understand what a proper lumbar lordosis should feel like, roll up a hand towel, stand with your back against the wall with your knees bent slightly, and place the rolled towel between the wall and your back, using your back to hold it in place.

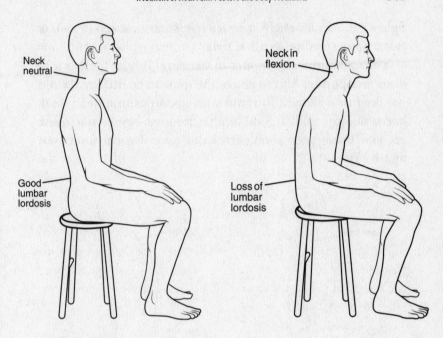

Neck
neutral

Good
lumbar
lordosis

Neck in
flexion

Loss of
lumbar
lordosis

Figures 23 and 24
Sitting postures. Figure 23 is good sitting posture with proper lumbar curve and neck upright. Figure 24 is poor sitting posture with bad lumbar curve, chest slumped forward, which causes the head and neck to be forward.

To see how low back posture affects your neck, try this experiment. Sit up straight on a stool or chair. Hold a good lumbar lordosis, lift your chest up, move your chin slightly back but keep it parallel to the ground, and gently bring your shoulder blades toward each other. This is the correct neck posture, and you can see how it is based on a solid lumbar foundation (figure 23). Now let your low back slump, and note the effect of the loss of the lumbar lordosis on your neck and head. They have now moved forward and out of balance (see figure 24). *This slouched posture is a significant cause of neck pain in people who sit for long periods of time.*

The same principle applies to standing. Proper lumbar lordosis is important for the rest of the spine to be balanced while standing or walking. To stand with good posture, bend your knees slightly, hold a good lumbar lordosis, bring your chest up, and bring your shoulder blades toward each other (see figure 25).

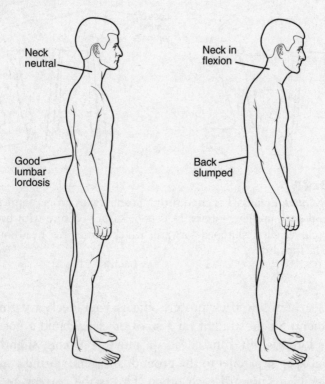

Figures 25 and 26
Standing posture. Figure 25 shows good standing posture with the lumbar curve maintained and the head and neck in neutral position. Figure 26 shows slumped posture with low back slumped, chest sunken, which causes the head and neck to be pushed forward.

THE NECK, CHEST, AND SHOULDERS

Good posture of the head and neck requires good posture of the chest and upper back, which in turn rest on the foundation provided by the lumbar spine. The position for your chest and upper back is simple: chest up, shoulders back, shoulder blades retracted (pulled back) toward each other slightly. To complete the proper alignment (see figure 25), pull your chin back slightly. This posture, called the neutral spine, should be used for sitting, standing, walking, and all activities of daily life. Although it may feel awkward at first, the more you use the neutral spine position, the more comfortable and balanced it will feel. When this position becomes automatic, your neck pain will usually begin to diminish.

Another way to help you picture the neutral spine posture was proposed by Dr. David Fardon in his book *Free Yourself from Neck Pain and Headache*. He recommends picturing a string attached to the top of your skull. Imagine that this string is being pulled upward toward the ceiling gently but steadily. As "the string" is pulled, your spine straightens, your neck feels longer, your head draws back, and your shoulders retract. In this neutral spine position, there is much less tension in your muscles because they do not have to work as hard to hold the balanced posture.

Bending Your Head Forward and Backward

When you are in the neutral spine position, it is easier to bend and turn your head and neck properly. You can bend your head and neck forward (flexion), backward (extension), rotate around the central axis (axial rotation), bend left and right (side bending), and do combination movements. When your neck is in the neutral position, turning or bending your head places less stress on the discs and facet joints.

Two of the worst positions for your neck are craning up and back (as in changing a lightbulb above your head), or bending too far forward (as in staying hunched over a book on a table that is too low). One good way to work overhead or below the knees while maintaining good mechanics is to imagine a "cervical strike zone." In baseball, the strike zone is the area that extends from just below the shoulders to the top of the knees. In proper neck mechanics, the cervical strike zone extends from your eyes to the tips of your fingers when your arms are hanging at your sides. To work overhead, you can move your cervical strike zone upward by standing on a secure stool or ladder, thus putting the task at eye level. To work closer to the ground, you need to lower your cervical strike zone by bending your knees, but keeping a good lumbar lordosis.

When bending your head forward or backward within the strike zone, the best technique is to use the "skull hinge." When using the skull hinge, the axis for bending is at the base of the skull, where it joins the top of your neck (figure 27). Picture the base of your skull as a hinged joint. The middle and lower parts of your neck should not bend. To get a feel for the skull hinge, look down slowly toward the floor, bending at the base of your skull, and keeping your chin retracted. Concentrate on keeping the rest of your neck from moving. Feel the motion occur at the axle or hinge at the top of your neck. Practice nodding your head using the skull hinge. As you lower your chin to your chest, you may feel some resistance, but it is rare to ever need to touch your chin to your chest.

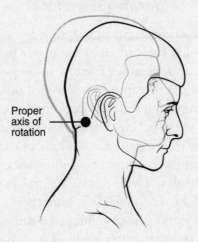

Figures 27 and 28

"Skull hinge." Figure 27 shows the head and neck bending forward with the proper axis of rotation. Figure 28 shows the head bending forward at the improper axis of rotation.

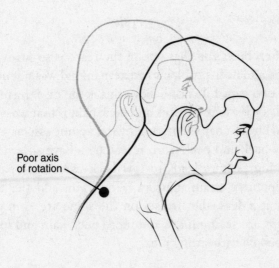

Turning Your Head

Try another experiment. Sit in a slumped position with your shoulders rounded forward and your upper back "collapsed." Your head will jut forward in front of your chest. Try turning your head to either side from this slumped position. You may feel and hear crunching and feel the limitation of motion.

Now return to the balanced neutral spine position by sitting up straight and restoring the normal lumbar curve in your low back, lifting your chest, and gently pulling back your shoulders and shoulder blades. Then, in this neutral position, turn to the left and right. It should feel smoother, easier, and less "crunchy" than turning from a slumped posture.

An even better way to turn your head to the left or right is to actually rotate your entire body as a unit. This is not usually practical, unless you have a chair with a swivel seat. An alternative is to rotate your upper body as a single unit at the hips, just below the waist. There is no rotation at the head or neck, and there is less stress on the low back as well.

SITTING

It has often been said that one of the reasons so many people have back and neck problems is that mankind was not meant to walk on two legs. I do not believe this is the case. Instead, one of the major reasons for back and neck pain is that we were not meant to sit on chairs! Although we may not associate sitting with low back and neck pain, researchers have shown us that poor sitting posture leads to low back pain, neck pain, and other repetitive strain injuries. When you add the tasks of working at a desk, the stresses on the spine are even greater. Physicians are seeing more and more neck pain and low back pain in people with sitting jobs.

I have briefly discussed sitting earlier, but the subject is so important that it is worth repeating some of the relevant concepts. The optimal position for the lumbar spine is a gentle curve in the shape of a C (the lumbar lordosis) that bends inward toward the belly button. Good posture for the chest, upper back, neck, and head require a good lumbar lordosis. Hold your chest up, slightly retract your shoulders, and bring your shoulder blades gently toward each other. This position allows your head and neck to rest comfortably over your shoulders. To complete the proper alignment (figure 23), hold your chin parallel to the floor and pulled back slightly.

In her book *The Chair*, the architect Galen Cranz recommends perching rather than sitting. Perching is a posture that is between sitting and standing. It requires a seat height of about twenty-four inches (the approximate height of a barstool). This is higher than most standard chairs, which have a seat height of seventeen to eighteen inches. You "perch" on the edge of the stool with your weight divided so that about 60 percent is on the buttocks area and 20 percent is on each foot. Your knees should be lower than your hips. The angle of your hip joint should be between 120 degrees and 135 degrees (figure 29). The perched position makes it difficult to round your back and requires you to use your back muscles for support. It promotes an expanded chest, retracted shoulders, and good head and neck position. Although perching on a high stool is good ergonomic posture, it may become impractical to use the desks and tables in most offices and homes.

A way to overcome poor ergonomic furniture design is to use a traditional chair as a perch. You perch on the edge of an ordinary chair that is against a wall so it cannot move, while kneeling on one knee on a pad on the floor and the other knee bent at 90 degrees (figure 30). Your weight should be distributed so that about 60 percent is on your buttocks, 30 percent

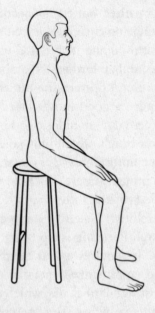

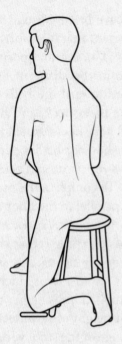

Figures 29 and 30

Perching. Figure 29 shows perching on a tall stool. The hip angle is about 120 degrees, and the body weight is divided equally between both feet and the butt. Figure 30 shows perching on a short stool or chair. One knee is on a pad on the ground. The body weight is divided equally between one knee, one foot, and the butt.

on the knee on the floor, and 10 percent on the other foot. When your knee gets sore, change to the other knee. Perched sitting on an ordinary chair can be used in restaurants, at home, or in an office.

An alternative to perching on a high stool or ordinary chair is to use a kneeling chair (also called a Balans chair), which was designed to accommodate the perched position but would fit under a standard desk or table. The original Balans chair has rocker bottoms that encourage motion and good padding for the knees, but it is expensive. Less-expensive versions sacrifice the rocker bottoms and good padding and are less comfortable. High-quality versions of kneeling chairs are offered by Back Saver and other companies.

Some people do not find the kneeling chair comfortable. An alternative is to use a seat that is designed in the shape of a saddle. When it is adjusted to the proper height, your knees will form the proper angle with your hips, you will sit up straight, and your legs will be apart slightly. Body weight can be shared between your butt region and both feet. "Saddle seats" are available commercially. You can also convert a stool to a saddle seat by rolling up a blanket and placing it with the ends of the column facing forward and backward on top of the stool.

Another technique to improve sitting posture is to raise your desk and use a bar stool or high kitchen stool. A drafting table with adjustable height makes a great desk. It has a large surface area, and the angle of the top surface can be adjusted. Some people can work in a recliner like the one made by Back Saver. A recliner supports the low back, supports the head, and reduces the load on your spine. There is an adjustable chair-side table and a lap desk that work well with a recliner to provide a functional work surface.

STANDING AND BENDING

Since your back and neck are part of an integrated system, your standing posture also influences the stresses placed on your neck. Proper standing posture, which is described above (figure 25), requires slightly bent knees, a good lumbar curve, an elevated chest, and slightly retracted shoulders.

To bend correctly without stressing your neck or low back, keep a good lumbar lordosis and bend forward at the hip joint. This is called a flat back bend. The axis of rotation is the hip joint or the "hip hinge." Do not round your low back. Keep your chest up and avoid bending at your neck. The motion should be at the hip joint, not the back. To get closer to the ground, bend your knees more. Once again, it will take time for bending properly to feel automatic and comfortable. However, again, there will be long-term rewards.

Lifting is best performed by bending at the knees, keeping the back straight, and looking forward, perhaps using a neck hinge if you need to look down (figure 31). If you round your back, your neck will follow into flexion, which is bad for your entire spine (figure 32).

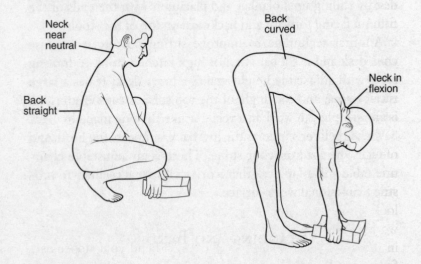

Figures 31 and 32
Lifting positions. Figure 31 shows lifting properly using a squat technique. The back is straight and the head and neck are neutral. Figure 32 shows lifting poorly with a rounded low back, rounded upper back, which forces the head and neck forward.

SPECIAL SITUATIONS

Desk Work

Sitting at a desk properly is much more difficult than it might seem, and presents a major ergonomic challenge. Some of the factors that contribute to sitting posture include the desk chair, the desk itself, the computer keyboard and monitor, and the size of the person who is sitting. Most variables can be adjusted to minimize the negative impact of desk work.

Sitting properly has been discussed above. There are many "ergonomic chairs" to aid sitting tolerance and posture, but most people do not take advantage of the chair design. Desk workers usually do not use the back of the chair for support and instead slump forward toward the desk. Your chair may be too low or the desk too high to encourage good posture. However, when well fitted and properly used, ergonomic chairs are quite helpful. If a kneeling chair is not appropriate for your needs, a good desk chair may solve the problem. It is preferable to purchase an ergonomic desk chair from a company that specializes in them. It is also important to sit in the chair at a desk before buying it, so it is advisable to buy it from a store rather than a catalog.

Depending on proper or improper use, the height and angle of your writing surface can either relieve or create neck pain (figures 33 and 34). Adjust your work surface to allow you to sit up straight, keep your head and neck directly over your shoulders, look straight ahead, and bend at the base of the skull. If your work surface is too low, you may find yourself tending to slump in the low back, round your shoulders, bend your upper back forward, and stick your neck forward, which places excess strain on the neck and low back. One solution is to use an adjustable-height drafting table or a fixed-height standing desk. Another alternative is to raise a conventional desk to the desired height by putting it on blocks.

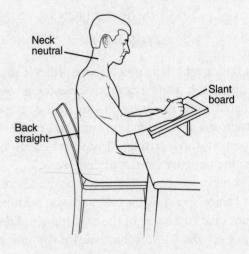

Figures 33 and 34

Sitting at a desk. Figure 33 shows sitting properly using a slant board, keeping the back straight, and the head and neck neutral. Figure 34 shows sitting poorly with low back rounded, shoulders rounded, which forces the head and neck forward.

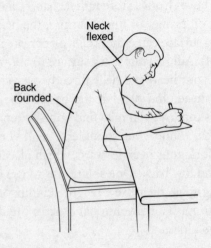

The best height for your desk is determined by the height of your seat. If you are doing keyboard entry, the optimal position is with your arms dangling at your sides and your elbows forming right angles when your hands are on the keyboard. If you do much more writing than keyboarding, the desk should be an inch or so higher. A functional compromise is to have a piece of plastic or smooth wood to place on your desk for writing. In addition, there should be enough room under your desk for your legs to be able to move around comfortably. Sometimes, drawers below the writing surface impinge on the free space below the desk, and may need to be removed.

The angle of the writing surface can be adjusted by raising the back of the desk more than the front. A slant board (figure 33), which is a portable surface that you place on the desk, works well to provide the best working angle and will hold books, papers, and keyboard. As mentioned above, the keyboard should be adjusted to allow you to work with both elbows at right angles while "typing." If the desk is too high, a keyboard tray attached under the top surface of the desk will lower it.

You may also have to change some work patterns. To avoid the detriments of staying in one position for hours at a time, take a five-minute break every hour or two. Get up, move around, stretch, and then return to work. If you try to vary your tasks, this will encourage frequent changes in position.

Many people feel they cannot devote this amount of time for neck pain prevention. However, if the minutes lost from work prevent or relieve pain, they will pay dividends by improving your efficiency, productivity, and the quality of your work, and by decreasing the number of workdays you will lose due to pain. It may seem excessive to devote thirty to forty minutes to your spine each workday. But doing the math can help you see the benefits of this time investment. For instance, every day of work that is missed has 480 lost minutes in it (8 hours times 60 minutes). That is equivalent to twelve full days of breaks! So you can see that in the long run, putting a little forethought and planning into "working smart" can pay off.

Your computer monitor should be placed directly in front of you, not at an angle. If you have a narrow desk, you may be tempted to put the monitor off to one side. This is a very awkward position that forces you to turn your upper body and neck. If your desk is too narrow, move it away from the wall to provide the necessary space. The height of the monitor should be adjusted so your eyes fall naturally on the middle of the screen.

When you are working from source material such as a text or notes, take care to position them properly. The best positions are between the keyboard and the monitor, propped up on a slant board, or held at eye level next to the screen by an attachable paper holder. Avoid placing the source material on the desk off to either side, since this will cause you to rotate and flex your head and neck.

Talking on the Telephone

A telephone headset is a must if you talk on the phone for long periods of time, especially if you write while you are talking. A headset eliminates the need to cradle the telephone between your ear and your shoulder, a terrible position for your neck. A speaker phone also works well, although some people find these rude and distant. In general, voice quality is better with headsets (see appendix B).

Driving and Your Neck

Many people find that being stuck in heavy traffic or driving for long distances is a pain in the neck and causes a pain in the neck. Many variables can be altered to minimize the strains on the neck. It is particularly important to have a good lumbar lordosis when you are sitting in a car seat. Some newer cars come with a built-in lumbar support. If this feature is not installed in your car, you can place a rolled towel in the small of the back. If the seat is too soft, you can purchase a back support to put directly on the car seat.

Raise the seat as high as possible to maximize the hip joint angle, and tilt it back to an angle that partially unloads the low back (30 degrees is ideal) but still allows a good view of the road. Adjust your head restraint to its maximum height, so that your head leans against it while you are driving. If the head restraint feels too far back, secure a small pillow to the restraint to close the gap between it and your head.

Get a large rearview mirror and add stick-ons for the side mirrors to increase your field of vision and minimize the need to turn your head. When you need to look left or right, try to do it while keeping your head against the head restraint, and when changing lanes or backing up, move your whole body around to get a good look.

Sleeping

People with chronic neck pain may sleep poorly because of the pain or because of depression that arises from the pain and impairment (see chapters 16 and 17). Some people have difficulty falling asleep, while others wake up frequently during the night. In either case, sleep is not restorative. When people awaken with increased neck pain, they may attribute it to "sleeping wrong."

Sleep posture is a difficult problem, because even when the bed is prepared for maximum support, the normal twisting and turning during the night causes pillows and neck supports to move. Sleep specialists have learned that most people have a preferred position in which they spend most of the night. Therefore, it can be useful to set up your bed to provide maximum support for this position. If you sleep primarily on your back, place a cylinder roll or pillow under your neck and a flat pillow under your head so the overall alignment of the neck and spine is neutral (figure 35). If your pillow is too high, it will place your neck into too much flexion (figure 36). If you sleep on your side, place a larger-diameter pillow under your neck and a smaller-diameter pillow under your head so the overall neck alignment is straight (figure 37) rather than curved (figure 38). With some people, a pillow placed under the waist improves alignment further. Check your sleeping posture with a mirror or a bedmate.

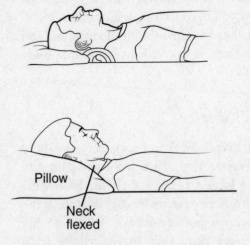

Figures 35 and 36
Neck rest position for sleeping on your back. Figure 35 shows proper sleep posture with a small pillow or rolled towel that supports the neck. Figure 36 shows a pillow that is too large and forces the head and neck into flexion.

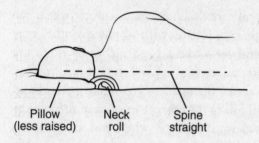

Pillow
(less raised)

Neck
roll

Spine
straight

Figures 37 and 38

Sleeping on your side. Figure 37 shows proper posture with a straight spine and a rolled towel or small pillow under the neck. Figure 38 shows poor posture with a curved spine because the pillow is too large.

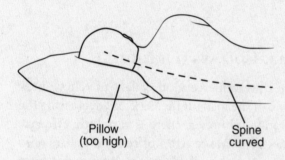

Pillow
(too high)

Spine
curved

Advertisements for neck pillows have increased in recent years, and all claim to have the best product. Researchers have compared pillows to see whether they help neck pain. One study compared each person's regular pillow to a cervical roll and a water pillow with respect to pain level in the morning, overall pain relief, and quality of sleep. The water pillow was superior to both the participants' own pillows and the cervical roll. There was less morning pain and improved quality of sleep with the water pillow.

The neck support pillows designed for air or car travel can help some people. One type inflates with air and the other type is filled with grain and feels like a beanbag. Both types are horseshoe-shaped and tend to stay in place, but, if not, you can sew a piece of Velcro across the open end to create a doughnut.

Your mattress should have the correct amount of firmness to keep your spine in a neutral position when you are lying on your side. When side lying, if the mattress is too firm, the shoulders and hips will take the pressure and force the lumbar spine to sag, putting your entire spine out of alignment. If the mattress is too soft, there will also be excess sagging. There is no evidence that a firm mattress is best, and contrary to popular opinion, too soft may be better than too hard. Your best bet is to purchase a mattress that can be returned if it is not satisfactory.

Neck Collars (Orthoses)

Doctors sometimes prescribe cervical collars to relieve neck pain by taking some of the load off the neck and decreasing the neck's range of motion. However, there is very little evidence that cervical collars help. Many types of cervical collars (also called cervical orthoses) are available, ranging from soft foam collars to hard plastic devices. The orthoses prescribed most often are the Philadelphia collar, the Miami-J collar, and the Malibu collar.

All collars restrict motion to some extent, and the stiffer the collar, the greater the restriction. Soft foam collars do not restrict forward bending (flexion) or backward bending (extension) sufficiently to do anything meaningful. All other collars are better. The Philadelphia collar is made of Styrofoam. It is lightweight, easy to fit, easy to use, inexpensive, and provides a small degree of restriction. Some spine specialists feel the best collar is the Miami-J collar, which is made of hard plastic. It is easy to fit, fairly comfortable, and immobilizes the neck well.

There are several circumstances when cervical collars might be used. They can be helpful as a part of neck first aid by immobilizing the neck to allow the person to function normally. They also may help people who, despite physical therapy and body mechanics training, continue to get increased pain after specific activities, such as gardening or prolonged driving. In these cases, an orthosis can be used during the activity to possibly prevent the flare. A cervical collar can also be a valuable teaching tool. By keeping your head and neck in the correct position during activities, the collar can "teach" you the feeling of proper neck positioning that you might not have learned from physical therapy and ergonomic training. I often refer to a cervical collar used for this purpose as "training wheels for your neck." Then, after a few months of using the collar, you will have learned the proper neck positions, and the collar will no longer be necessary.

Some physicians object to the routine use of cervical collars, because, in theory, using a collar may weaken your muscles because the collar does part of their work. To overcome this problem, you must do strengthening exercises. In fact, some people who flare when exercising do better if they routinely wear the orthoses when exercising. In addition, a cervical collar may identify the wearer as an injured person, and this might have negative psychological implications.

10
Treatment of Neck Pain: Medications

The use of medications to treat most of the common ailments of our society is widespread, and the treatment of pain is no exception. The search for relief of chronic and severe pain leads most people to try medications at some time. We are constantly barraged with television and magazine advertisements that suggest miraculous relief from over-the-counter medications. Each manufacturer claims to have the best drug or "the pain reliever doctors prescribe most." It is important to keep in mind that although medications never cure neck pain, they can often reduce it enough to allow you to exercise more aggressively and maintain your activity levels. In chronic neck pain, the proper medications can also improve quality of life considerably.

In this chapter, I present an overview of the prescription and over-the-counter medications used most often for acute and chronic pain. In addition to the pure pain relievers, other medication may play a role in the treatment of neck pain. Accordingly, anti-inflammatory medications, sleeping pills, antidepressants, muscle relaxants, and other medications are also discussed in this chapter. This information is intended only to be a guide, and it is always best to consult your physician for specific recommendations. It is also important to see your doctor if you are using high doses of over-the-counter medications such as ibuprofen (Motrin, Advil, and others) or naproxen (Aleve) and the pain is not improving.

Medications that relieve pain are called analgesics. Different analgesics act at different sites along the pain pathway. Some work at the site of injury (peripherally acting analgesics) and others act on pain centers in the brain and spinal cord (centrally acting analgesics). Aspirin (Bayer, Anacin, and others), acetaminophen (Tylenol), and ibuprofen are peripherally acting analgesics available over the counter. Stronger medications require a prescription. The centrally acting analgesics are the narcotics, more properly called opioid analgesics. They all share similar chemical structures with opium. Some occur naturally in nature, but those used pharmacologically are usually synthetic. The opioids are more potent than the peripherally acting analgesics, and are used for moderate to severe pain. Codeine and morphine are two centrally acting analgesics.

Pain medications can be taken in two different ways: when pain occurs (called pain-contingent dosing), or on a fixed schedule to prevent pain from occurring or getting worse (time-contingent dosing). The goal of pain-contingent dosing is to reduce pain that is already present, while the goal of time-contingent dosing is to keep pain under control. Pain-contingent dosing is best for pain that occurs only periodically, such as when you take aspirin or ibuprofen for a headache. Time-contingent dosing works best for chronic or severe pain that is expected to last for several days or weeks. If the pain problem is bad enough to require time-contingent dosing, most people should be under the care of a physician. However, even with time-contingent dosing, occasional pain-contingent "rescue" doses may be necessary when pain worsens.

Peripherally Acting Analgesics

There are two categories of peripherally acting analgesics: acetaminophen and nonsteroidal anti-inflammatory drugs, or NSAIDs for short. In turn, there are two categories of NSAIDs, aspirin and the nonaspirin NSAIDs. Aspirin, ibuprofen, and naproxen are the NSAIDs that are available over the counter. Stronger ones require a prescription. There are more than a dozen NSAIDs available, some of which are listed in table 5. It is not clear whether prescription NSAIDs provide better pain relief than ibuprofen, but they are more convenient to take and probably have fewer side effects. There are also medications that combine acetaminophen or aspirin with caffeine to improve pain relief.

Table 5
Some of the Many NSAIDs

Generic Name	Brand Name	Class**
Ibuprofen*	Motrin, Advil	Short-acting
Naproxen*	Naprosyn, Naprelan	Short to intermediate
Diclofenac	Voltaren, Cataflam	Short-acting
Etodolac	Lodine	Short to intermediate
Oxaprozin	Daypro	Long-acting
Nabumetone	Relafen	Long-acting
Rofecoxib	Vioxx	Long-acting
Celecoxib	Celebrex	Long-acting

* Low-dose sizes available over the counter. Higher-dose sizes by prescription.
** See text for explanations.

Mechanisms of Action

The way a drug works in the body is called its mechanism of action, and we do not completely understand the mechanism of action for the analgesic effect of the NSAIDs or acetaminophen. We do know the NSAIDs inhibit inflammation, which is defined as the presence of tenderness, redness, and swelling. Inflammation is the end result of a series of biochemical reactions that occur after injury that depend in part on the action of an enzyme called cyclooxygenase, or COX for short. NSAIDs inhibit COX and thereby decrease inflammation and pain.

However, the anti-inflammatory action does not fully explain the mechanism of action of NSAIDs. It can take seven to ten days for the anti-inflammatory effect to occur, but when you take NSAIDs, pain relief may occur in less than an hour. This is much sooner than any decrease in inflammation could occur, which implies that analgesia has other mechanisms besides the inhibition of COX.

Types of NSAIDs

There is no best NSAID. In a given individual, one may work better than another despite the fact that all NSAIDs appear to do the same things biochemically, and there is no way to predict which one is best for each person. To help choose an NSAID, it is useful to divide them into three groups based on how quickly they work and how long they last (tables 5 and 6). The short-acting NSAIDs begin to work in thirty to sixty minutes and provide relief for six to eight hours. The intermediate-acting drugs take twice as long to work, but may last up to twelve hours. The long-acting NSAIDs may take several hours to begin to work, but last up to twenty-four hours.

The short and intermediate NSAIDs are better choices for

acute pain or flares of chronic pain, when pain-contingent dosing is used. The long-acting drugs are preferred for chronic pain when there is a need for time-contingent dosing. If your pain appears to be related to inflammation, your doctor may advise one of the long-acting drugs.

Aspirin

Aspirin has been used for almost one hundred years, and even today it remains a reasonable choice for mild to moderate pain. It is available without prescription and it is very inexpensive. In addition to providing pain relief, aspirin has an anti-inflammatory effect when used every eight hours for several days or weeks. However, using aspirin for long periods increases the incidence of side effects, especially stomach irritation, and that is one reason why the other NSAIDs are used much more often.

One adult tablet contains 325 mg of aspirin, which is the lowest effective dose. There is additional pain relief as the dose is increased up to a maximum of 1,000 mg. There is no difference in effectiveness between different brands of aspirin. The "name brands" such as Bayer, Excedrin, or Anacin are more expensive, but they have a longer shelf life. Generic brands are less expensive, but do not last as long when stored. If you use aspirin only occasionally, it is cost-effective to buy a small quantity of a name brand. If you intend to use aspirin regularly, it is best to buy large quantities of the least-expensive brand. If you notice that the contents of your aspirin bottle smell like vinegar, this means the tablets may be getting old and should be replaced.

Other NSAIDs

In order to decrease side effects and increase effectiveness, NSAIDs that do not contain aspirin were developed. Ibuprofen was the first nonaspirin NSAID, and it is now available over the counter. Newer NSAIDs appear to have fewer side effects and are more convenient because some are effective taken only once per day. As I have alluded to earlier, one of the puzzling things about these drugs is that although they all do the same thing biochemically, people respond to them differently. Some patients respond to one NSAID but not another, and some people experience side effects with one NSAID but not others. It may be helpful to keep this in mind so that you do not become discouraged if the first NSAID is not effective, but your doctor wants to try different ones. Table 6 lists some of the more commonly used NSAIDs, their minimally effective doses, the expected duration of relief, and the approximate dose necessary for anti-inflammatory benefits.

Table 6

Nonsteroidal Anti-inflammatory Drugs.
Dose Sizes, Duration of Relief, and Anti-inflammatory Doses

Drug	OTC Size (mg)	Pill Sizes (mg)	Usual Dose (mg)	Duration of Relief (hours)	Anti-inflammatory Dose (mg per day)
Ibuprofen*	200	400 600 800	400 3 to 4 times per day	6 to 8	1,800 to 2,400
Naproxen*	275	250 375 500	250 2 or 3 times per day	8 to 12	550 to 1,000
Relafen	N/A	500 750	1,000 to 1,500 once daily	24	1,000
Daypro	N/A	600	1,200 once daily	24	1,200
Voltaren	N/A	50 75	50 to 75 3 times per day	8	150

(continued)

Table 6 (continued)

Drug	OTC Size (mg)	Pill Sizes (mg)	Usual Dose (mg)	Duration of Relief (hours)	Anti-inflammatory Dose (mg per day)
Lodine	N/A	400 500 600	200 to 400 3 times per day	8	600
Vioxx	N/A	12.5 25 50	12.5 to 25 once daily	24	12.5 to 25
Celebrex	N/A	100 200	200 to 400 daily	24	100 to 400

* Approved for up to 5 days' use for acute pain.

Side Effects of Aspirin and Other NSAIDs

The NSAIDs have an impressive list of possible side effects, ranging from stomach irritation to liver and kidney damage with long-term use. But considering how frequently they are used, NSAIDs are actually relatively safe. In fact, aspirin, ibuprofen, and naproxen are considered safe enough to be available without prescription. In general, the risk of side effects from NSAIDs increases at higher doses and with longer use. Most side effects are minor and disappear promptly when you stop taking the drug, but a few can be serious. Therefore, particularly with long-term use, the risk of side effects must be weighed against the degree of pain relief. It is not possible to predict who will experience side effects, but people with previous ulcers, bad heartburn, the elderly, and people with serious medical conditions such as liver, kidney, or heart disease are more likely to develop problems.

The most common side effects of NSAIDs are abdominal pain and heartburn. NSAIDs block production of some of the protective mucous coating of the intestine, so the lining of the esophagus (food pipe), stomach, or duodenum (first part of the small intestine) can become irritated or inflamed. It is a systemic effect of the drug, not merely the direct contact of the pill with the stomach lining. People who experience the abdominal pain often describe it as a gnawing or burning sensation in the pit of the stomach. Ulcers are much less common, but can be serious, because ulcers may bleed or penetrate the lining of the stomach or duodenum. Therefore, the decision to continue taking an NSAID when you have abdominal pain must be made carefully in conjunction with your physician. If the NSAID provides excellent pain relief, but causes stomach or esophageal side effects, you have options available to you. It is reasonable to try a different NSAID to see if you can get equally good relief without side effects. Another option that your doctor may suggest is to treat the symptoms with a medication, such as Prilosec, that blocks stomach acid production. However, if the NSAID is providing only marginal benefit, then the drug should be stopped. The newer NSAIDs, Vioxx and Celebrex, are less likely to cause stomach or intestinal side effects.

On rare occasions, NSAIDs can cause liver damage, usually without symptoms until the damage is serious. Therefore, anyone taking NSAIDs long-term, needs to have blood tests done every six to twelve months to detect any damage at an early stage because the liver will usually heal if the NSAID is stopped at that point.

Long-term use of NSAIDs can also cause kidney problems, the most common of which are water and salt retention with swelling of the ankles (edema). The swelling is not usually dangerous, but if it is severe or keeps getting worse, it can be a sign of more serious kidney damage, and it is important to see a doctor. The NSAIDs can also cause serious kidney problems, but, again, these are usually reversible if detected early. A good precaution for anyone taking NSAIDs for more than a few months is to have blood tests done every six to twelve months.

NSAIDs can also interfere with the function of platelets, the cells in your blood that are essential for the clotting process that stops bleeding. Some people are more susceptible to clotting problems than others. Once again, the newer NSAIDs, such as Vioxx and Celebrex, are less likely to cause these platelet problems. Clotting problems can be dangerous if you are having surgery or need an invasive medical procedure. That is why your doctor will ask whether you are taking these medications when he or she is planning to do surgery. The risk can be minimized by stopping the NSAIDs for five days before any invasive procedure

CENTRALLY ACTING ANALGESICS (OPIOID OR NARCOTIC ANALGESICS)

The centrally acting analgesics are the opioids, also referred to as narcotics. Opioids act on the major pain centers in the brain and spinal cord to relieve pain. Most opioids are potent analgesics, but a few are no stronger than the NSAIDs. In general, the degree of pain relief increases as the dose is increased, but so do the side effects. During episodes of acute pain, opioids can be administered by injection or by mouth. To treat chronic pain, opioids usually are administered either by mouth or through a patch placed on the skin (transdermal patch). Table 7 is a list of the opioids used most commonly for chronic pain.

The relief of pain is one of the primary goals of medicine, and the opioids are powerful drugs in that regard. When used correctly in the right patient, opioids can provide significant pain relief with just a few side effects and little risk. However, in the wrong patient or for the wrong condition, opioids may not relieve pain and can cause serious side effects or complications.

The use of opioids to treat pain due to cancer or severe acute pain is not controversial. However, physicians disagree about the use of opioid analgesics for chronic pain not due to cancer. Until recently, most doctors would not prescribe opioid analgesics for chronic pain, unless it was due to cancer. They feared opioids would cause addiction, severe side effects, and organ damage. In addition, opioids are controlled substances regulated by the Drug Enforcement Administration (DEA). In six states, copies of prescriptions written for opioid analgesics go to the state, and doctors may fear that prescribing opioids for people with chronic pain might put their medical licenses in jeopardy.

However, over the last five to ten years, this thinking has been changing. Research has been presented that demonstrates the usefulness of opioids as one part of a pain-management program and government agencies are becoming more enlightened about the use of opioids to treat pain. As a result, it is now considered good medical care to use opioid analgesics for chronic pain in patients who are carefully selected as being likely candidates for success. Opioids appear to be most useful in patients in whom all other means of pain treatment have been exhausted, whose pain markedly interferes with their quality of life, and who have a clear but not otherwise treatable explanation for the pain. Before prescribing opioids, physicians should make sure that the patient does not have a history of addictive disease and is psychologically healthy. Anyone taking opioids for chronic pain must be followed carefully, usually by a pain medicine specialist.

It has been shown that opioid analgesics can be effective and have minimal side effects in many, but not all patients. However, there are potential problems with the long-term use of opioid analgesics. Obviously, opioids do not cure the problem; they cover it up. Therefore, they are appropriate only if the problem cannot be cured directly. They are a treatment for life, and just as diabetics must take insulin for life to control their blood sugars, pain patients who respond to opioids will most likely need them for life.

Most patients who take opioids will have side effects. Nausea and slight sedation are common at the beginning of treatment, but usually get better over time. Interestingly, difficulties with thinking, problems concentrating, or bad coordination rarely occur when patients are on constant doses of opioids. However, at the beginning of treatment and when doses are increased, these side effects may be present, but they gradually disappear as treatment continues. Constipation usually is a chronic side effect, and requires laxatives such as Senokot, dioctyl sodium sulfate (DSS), and drinking plenty of fluids. Other side effects include itching, sweating, and occasionally loss of sexual desire (libido), which may be due to opioids lowering the levels of the hormone testosterone. If this is the reason, the testosterone can be replaced by means of a transdermal patch.

Almost all patients who take opioids for weeks or months will become dependent on them, a fact that frightens many people who might be considering long-term opioid therapy. The stigma attached to opioids remains very strong in our culture, and has led to confusion about dependence, addiction, and the use of opioids for pain control. Dependence means that the body has gotten used to a drug, and if the drug were stopped suddenly, the patient would go through drug withdrawal. The severity, type, and duration of withdrawal symptoms vary greatly from person to person, and depend on the individual person as well as the drug's potency and duration of use. Dependence is not the same as addiction. Addiction means continued use of a drug or substance despite harm. One hallmark of addiction is loss of control. Addiction and dependence are discussed in more detail in chapter 16, The Psychology of Pain.

Table 7

Some Opioid Analgesics (Narcotics) Used Most Often for Chronic Pain

Chemical Name	Brand Name	Comments
Morphine	MS Contin Oramorph	Expect 8- to 12-hour relief
Oxycodone	Roxycodone* Oxycontin	Percocet is oxycodone plus acetaminophen
Methadone	Dolophine	Very inexpensive
Fentanyl	Duramorph	Absorbed through skin New patch every 2 to 3 days
Levorphanol	Levo-Dromoran	Small dose size may mean taking many pills per day
Codeine*	Many	Short-acting Not good for chronic pain
Hydrocodone*	Vicodin Lortab Norco Zydone	Short-acting Not good for chronic pain

* Not a good choice for chronic pain. May be used as rescue doses for breakthrough pain.

When treating chronic pain, most pain specialists prefer to prescribe opioids that are released slowly but continuously from the intestine (MS Contin, Oramorph, Oxycontin, and others) or through the skin (Duragesic). Other good choices are the long-acting opioids such as methadone or levorphanol. The goal of using sustained release or long-acting opioids is to maintain a fairly constant level in the blood to keep pain under better control.

There is no best opioid and no dose that is correct for every patient, because some patients respond to one opioid and not another, and some patients need higher doses than others. The dose must be adjusted to find the best ratio of benefit to side effects. About two-thirds of well-selected patients with chronic pain will feel much better with opioid analgesics, and about 20 percent cannot tolerate the drugs. The use of opioid analgesics is a major commitment, and must be considered very carefully by both patient and doctor.

Muscle Relaxants

Muscle relaxants (table 8) are often prescribed for patients with neck pain, even though there are no good scientific studies to show these drugs relieve muscle spasm. Muscle relaxants do not select out muscles in spasm, but instead probably act on the brain to cause general relaxation throughout the body. Many doctors who specialize in pain medicine or addiction feel the muscle relaxants produce dependence, and withdrawal symptoms may occur when the drugs are stopped.

However, muscle relaxants have been on the market for so long, and they are so well named, that doctors and patients assume they are effective. I cannot recommend these drugs, except perhaps for two or three days if there is a flare of pain.

Table 8

Muscle Relaxants

Generic	Brand Name
Carisoprodol	Soma
Methocarbamol	Robaxin
Cyclobenzaprine	Flexeril
Baclofen	Lioresal
Orphenadrine	Norflex
Tizanidine	Zanaflex
Metaxalone	Skelaxin

SLEEPING PILLS

Many people with chronic neck pain have difficulty sleeping. Some people have difficulty falling asleep while others wake up frequently during the night. Either way, the result is that sleep is neither restful nor restorative. In people with neck pain, disturbed sleep can be caused by pain during the night, bad sleep posture, and depression.

In chapter 9, I discuss mattresses, pillows, and sleeping positions. By reading that chapter, you may be able to find a sleep position in which your neck is supported and your head, neck, and chest are kept in good alignment during the night. In turn, this may improve your sleep without the need for drugs.

Often, however, finding the right sleeping position is not enough. Many people with chronic pain need medications to sleep well. Several over-the-counter products, such as melatonin, are effective for some people. When over-the-counter medications fail, prescription sleeping pills may be indicated.

Most of these drugs are useful for the short-term treatment of insomnia, and if used one or two times per week, they usually are safe and effective. However, using sleeping pills more frequently diminishes their effectiveness, people tend to become dependent on them, and after a while they cannot sleep without them. In fact, some people who have been using sleeping pills regularly may get "rebound insomnia" and need progressively higher doses to sleep. None of the many sleeping pills on the market are perfect, and most will produce dependence. The sleeping pills used most often are shown in table 9. A newer drug, zolpidem (Ambien), has a different chemical structure and appears better, safer, and less likely to cause dependence and rebound insomnia.

For most patients with chronic neck pain and sleep difficulty, sedating-type antidepressant drugs are a better choice. They are reasonably safe, effective for sleep, and have the additional benefit of providing some pain relief as well.

Table 9
Sleeping Pills

Generic	Brand Name	Usual Dose (mg)
Zolpidem	Ambien	5 or 10
Temazepam	Restoril	15 or 30
Flurazepam	Dalmane	15 or 30
Diazepam	Valium	5 or 10
Triazolam	Halcion	0.25 or 0.5

ANTIDEPRESSANTS

There are three major reasons that antidepressants are prescribed for chronic pain: to improve pain, to treat depression, and to help with disturbed sleep. In chronic pain, the levels of some biochemicals, particularly norepinephrine, that help the body's natural pain relief system are often too low. This leads to a decrease in pain tolerance and worsening pain. One class of antidepressants, the tricyclic antidepressants, can help restore norepinephrine levels to normal, which may improve pain. The best antidepressants for pain relief are nortriptyline, amitriptyline, and desipramine. The doses of antidepressants needed for pain control are usually lower than those used to treat depression, and therefore there are fewer side effects (table 10). Antidepressants can help pain even in patients who are not depressed. The relief is not immediate, and may take up to three or four weeks.

Table 10

Some Antidepressants Useful for Chronic Pain

Generic	Brand	Value for Pain	Value for Depression	Value for Sleep
Nortriptyline	Pamelor	High	Medium	Medium
Amitriptyline	Elavil	High	Medium	High
Desipramine	Norpramin	High	Medium	Low
Venlafaxine	Effexor	Medium	Medium	Medium
Doxepin	Sinequan	Low	Medium	High
Trazodone	Desyrel	Low	Low	High
Fluoxetine	Prozac	Low	High	Low
Sertraline	Zoloft	Low	Medium	Low
Paroxetine	Paxil	Low	Medium	Low
Citalopram	Celexa	Low	High	Low
Mirtazapine	Remeron	Low	High	High

The newer antidepressants work on a different brain chemical, serotonin, and they belong to a class of drugs called selective serotonin reuptake inhibitors (SSRI). The SSRIs are very effective for depression, but not very good for the treatment of pain. However, many patients with chronic pain are depressed, and depression can make the pain worse, in which case the SSRIs can be useful. In some patients, SSRIs are combined with the tricyclic or other antidepressants to treat multiple symptoms.

When medications are necessary for sleep in patients with pain, the sedating antidepressant drugs are a better choice than sleeping pills. One of the side effects of tricyclic antidepressants is sedation, and we can use the sedation to help sleep while simultaneously treating pain and depression.

The starting dose for nortriptyline, amitriptyline, and desipramine is usually 10 mg. The dose is increased in increments of 10 mg every three to five days to a dose of about 50 mg. This level should be maintained for three or four weeks before increasing it. It takes several weeks at the higher doses for pain to improve.

All antidepressants have the potential to cause side effects, which are generally related to the class of the drug, the dose, the general age and health of the patient, and interactions with other drugs. The most common side effects of the tricyclic antidepressants are dry mouth, lowered blood pressure, sedation, constipation, and urinary retention, among others. The most common side effects of the SSRIs are nausea, weight loss, irritability, and decrease in sexual function. It is difficult to predict which patients will have which side effects, and it takes collaboration between doctor and patient to maximize the benefit and minimize the side effects.

11
Treatment of Neck Pain:
The Role of the Physician

Most people with neck pain never need to see a physician. However, when neck pain does not go away on its own or with self-care techniques, a well-qualified physician can offer useful advice, order diagnostic testing, and provide sophisticated treatment.

The majority of people with neck pain will respond to strength training, the use of proper body mechanics, and over-the-counter medications. People who do not improve may need professional care. Very often, a chiropractor or physical therapist can provide the additional help needed. Only about 10 percent of patients with chronic neck pain will require specialized testing, prescription medications, spinal injections, or surgery. However, if you need to see a medical doctor, it is important to choose the right doctor for you. Not all doctors have the same interest, training, and experience with neck pain.

Choosing a Doctor

When you are dealing with neck pain, especially if it is chronic, it is probably best to choose a doctor who specializes in the spine, but this is not always possible if you do not live in a major metropolitan area. Many doctors may take this common problem for granted and may not be aware of the most current information about diagnosis and treatment of neck pain and whiplash, which is published in specialty journals that are not usually read by primary care doctors.

Some specialists, such as neurosurgeons and orthopedists, face different problems. Their training was primarily hospital-based and dealt with patients who were in severe pain and were admitted to the hospital for pain control or surgery. Many of these specialists never received specialized training in nonsurgical care, rehabilitation, or medication use, and so may be unfamiliar with modern methods of nonsurgical treatment of neck pain.

On the other hand, spine specialists, many of whom belong to an organization called the North American Spine Society (NASS), devote their careers to the treatment of neck and back pain. These doctors are very likely to stay up to date by attending their society's yearly meetings, and reading published scientific findings in their specialty journals. Many large cities have private medical practices or university-based centers that specialize in spine problems. Specialists in sports medicine or rehabilitation (physiatrists) often have had advanced training in neck and back problems. When you call an office to make an appointment, inquire if the doctor has a special interest in spine problems and if he or she is a member of NASS. If you are not satisfied with the information you receive or your progress after a few visits, consider getting another opinion.

Some people belong to health maintenance organizations that do not allow you to choose your own specialist physician. You may have to rely on a referral from your primary care physician. However, you certainly are entitled to discuss your need for a referral with your doctor, and participate in the choice of specialist. This chapter (and the remainder of this book) will provide you with the information about what you should expect from a spine specialist. If you feel that your treatment is not being tailored to your needs, then you may need to request another consultation.

ROLES OF A DOCTOR

In this section, I outline the many things a physician does with regard to neck pain. For many people, their first contact with the medical system is with a primary care physician who will begin the evaluation and treatment. The primary doctor may refer you to physical therapy, prescribe medications, and, if you are not getting better, refer you to a specialist. If you respond, no further action is necessary, but, if not, the primary care doctor serves as the "gatekeeper," and makes any necessary referrals to a specialist.

Making a Diagnosis

A definitive diagnosis is not essential in the early stages of the treatment of neck pain, because most of the time, the pain gets better without specific treatment. However, if your pain does not improve, an accurate diagnosis makes it possible to plan more sophisticated treatment with spinal injections or occasionally surgery. I have previously discussed the possible causes of chronic neck pain (see chapter 2) and the details of evaluation (see chapter 3). It is your doctor's responsibility to order the necessary tests to make the diagnosis.

Medicine is an art based on science. At least in part, because it is an art, there are bound to be controversies. The biggest controversies in the field of neck pain are whether discs can cause pain when they are not pressing on nerves (discogenic pain) or the spinal cord, and whether facet joints cause pain. If your doctor does not consider the diagnosis of discogenic pain, he or she would not order discograms or, for severe pain, consider surgery. If your doctor does not believe that facet joints are a common cause of neck pain in whiplash, he or she would not recommend medial branch blocks or a neurotomy (see chapters 2 and 3). So part of the diagnostic process is based on the individual doctor's philosophy and belief system.

When neck pain is chronic, a specific diagnosis is important for several reasons. First of all, it may lead to specific treatment. Second, a specific diagnosis also gives the doctor an idea of the expected outcome for that particular problem, often referred to as the prognosis. This is important because many people with chronic pain worry about the future. Constantly dealing with pain makes them feel vulnerable, and they are often concerned they will get worse, not better. They worry that they will lose the use of an arm or become paralyzed. They might think that if the doctor is not able to say what is wrong, the doctor cannot know how to treat the problem, nor what the future holds. Part of the doctor's responsibility is to allay these fears about the future, and to reassure the patient that even if the pain is not relieved, there is much that can be done to restore and maintain function despite the pain.

Explaining the Diagnosis

A doctor is a teacher. Many doctors are experienced at teaching medical students or younger doctors in training. However, the major job of a doctor is to educate his or her own patients. An informed patient makes a better patient. Patients who understand their problems will participate fully in their treatment. They will understand the rationale behind the testing and the interpretation of the results. If fully informed about their condition, patients are also more likely to follow treatment instructions. It is the doctor's role to explain the diagnosis, the meaning of the diagnosis, the treatment plan, and the prognosis.

Sadly, in the current era of managed care and its emphasis on cost containment, the reimbursement for physicians has decreased substantially. Time becomes much more of a premium because doctors are reimbursed much less for the time they spend with each patient, despite the fact that it costs more to run an office. Some doctors compensate for the decreased payments by seeing more patients, but then there is less time for each. To overcome this time shortage, doctors can rely on books, printed handouts, other reference materials, or office staff specially trained in patient education to "fill the communication gap." However, it is still your doctor's job to be sure that you understand your problem.

Obtaining Consultation

No doctor can know everything, and all doctors will make mistakes in diagnosis and treatment. When a patient is not getting better, a good doctor obtains consultation from another doctor who may be more experienced with that particular problem. In patients with chronic neck pain, internists, family practitioners, general orthopedists, or even neurologists may not have the experience to help the patient, and should seek second opinions from specialists who can help.

Many patients with chronic pain become depressed. This increases their pain and decreases their ability to function. In some patients, a delay in the expected recovery may be due in part to psychological factors (see chapters 16 and 17). The primary doctor should obtain psychological or psychiatric consultation when he or she suspects that psychological factors are playing some role in the problem.

Prescribing Physical Therapy

Chapters 8 and 9 explain how strength and body mechanics training can lead to long-term improvement. Many patients do well with a self-directed program, but some need individualized professional instruction from a physical therapist (see chapter 13). Not all physical therapists provide this type of care. Some therapists emphasize "hands-on therapy," and may do only passive treatments, using spinal manipulation, heat, ultrasound, and massage. This is fine for symptom control, but unless these techniques are combined with strength and body mechanics training, they will not provide long-term benefit. It is the doctor's responsibility to refer patients to therapists who have the skills and knowledge to deliver the proper care. The doctor should also review the treatment program on a regular basis to be sure it is meeting the patient's needs.

Ordering Tests

Most people with neck pain do not need testing, but those who are not getting better usually do. There are many tests available to help diagnose neck pain, including X-rays, MRI scans,

CT scans, myelograms, EMG, and spinal injections (see chapter 3). It is the doctor's responsibility to decide which tests are appropriate and when they should be done. It is also the responsibility of the doctor to refer the patient for the highest-quality tests.

A physician uses several criteria to decide when to order testing and which tests to request, including the severity of the pain, duration of pain, and whether he or she has found evidence of nerve damage while doing the physical examination. The patient with mild or intermittent pain does not usually need to have testing. However, when pain increases, fails to respond to exercise and physical therapy, or begins to interfere with the activities of daily living, testing is indicated. Other indications for diagnostic testing include evidence of significant nerve damage on physical examination, or progression of nerve damage while the patient is undergoing treatment.

Usually, the first tests to be ordered are plain X-rays and an MRI scan. Many doctors just get an MRI, but because MRI only shows soft tissues, adding plain X-rays, which show bone, adds to the information. X-rays will also show if there is narrowing of the disc space, bone spurs, or perhaps some instability. An MRI will show disc degeneration, disc herniation, pressure on the spinal cord, and many other abnormalities if present.

Prescribing Medications

The role of medications in the management of many people with neck pain has been discussed in detail in chapter 10. As you know, the more powerful medications require a physician's prescription. It is important to remember that although medications can provide some degree of pain relief, they will not provide a cure for your spine problem.

THERAPEUTIC INJECTIONS

Most cervical spine problems improve with time, exercise, and use of good body mechanics. However, severe pain prevents some patients from being able to exercise or participate in body mechanics training. Such patients need more aggressive pain control to enable them to carry out a nonoperative treatment program and allow the injury to heal. Therapeutic cervical spine injections are part of a modern nonoperative treatment program.

In experienced hands, cervical spine injections are usually safe, but there is a very small risk of serious complications. Therefore, neck injections should only be performed by an experienced physician who has had special training in these techniques, and after X-rays and an MRI have been performed. These specialized neck injections should be done using "real-time X-rays" during the procedure (that is, imaging such as fluoroscopy done simultaneously to guide the physician's placement of the needle). Most patients experience little or no discomfort from the injections, but there is often some soreness at the injection site for a few days.

In both epidural injections and selective nerve root blocks, a long-acting form of cortisone is placed in the area of inflammation, usually Celestone or Decadron. When inflammation and swelling are reduced, pain usually improves, but injections never cure a spine problem. You may be concerned about the health risk associated with the use of steroid or cortisone injections. These risks are real, but the complications linked to steroids are much more common with their oral use over long periods of time in patients with serious medical conditions. Steroid spine injections appear safe if limited to three or four times per year.

Epidural Corticosteroid Injections

Epidural corticosteroid injections are probably the cervical spine injections performed most often. They work especially well for disc herniations and spinal stenosis (see chapters 2 and 3), and are usually more effective when you have symptoms of arm pain rather than neck pain. Pain relief usually lasts a few weeks and then the epidural injection can be repeated two or three times. Often, the duration of relief increases with each injection. In some patients, pain from disc herniations gets better over time. Therefore, if pain can be controlled with injections, the disc might heal, thus avoiding the need for surgery.

Selective Nerve Root Blocks (SNRB)

Selective nerve root blocks (SNRB) are also called transforaminal epidural injections. SNRB may provide relief from arm pain due to a disc herniation or narrowed nerve root canal (spinal stenosis), and is usually more effective for arm pain than neck pain. During an SNRB, the area around a single nerve is injected with a local anesthetic and long-acting corticosteroid to decrease the inflammation. In some patients, a series of two to four injections can help them avoid surgery. Selective nerve root injection may be recommended instead of standard epidural injection when the herniation is to one side, especially if the disc has herniated into the side canal (foramen). However, there are more complications with SNRB than epidurals, and they should be done by an experienced doctor.

Radiofrequency Neurotomy

Radiofrequency neurotomy will relieve the pain from facet joints in at least 70 percent of patients. When patients get short-term relief after two medial branch blocks (see chapter 3), radiofrequency neurotomy may be indicated. Pain relief usually lasts nine to eighteen months, and when relief fades, the neurotomy can be repeated.

To perform the procedure, an insulated needle connected to a radiofrequency generator is placed on the nerve. The needle is heated to coagulate the nerve, which then can no longer conduct pain signals. The procedure is safe in expert hands, but most patients feel worse immediately afterward, and it may be one to three weeks before they feel better.

Neck Surgery

Indications for Surgery

Except for a fractured neck after trauma such as a serious car accident, very few patients need emergency neck surgery. In very rare cases, a massive disc herniation can put pressure on the spinal cord, cause a loss of bowel or bladder function, and require urgent surgery, but most other indications for surgery are elective—that is, the surgery can be planned for and performed when you and your doctor choose.

Some indications for neck surgery are somewhat controversial. Almost all physicians agree that nerve root compression with severe arm pain or weakness and spinal cord compression are indications for surgery. In addition, most surgeons feel that patients with nerve root compression and moderate arm pain or muscle weakness that have not responded to aggressive conservative care most likely are also good candidates for surgery.

However, there is controversy about the role of surgery for neck pain when there is no evidence of pressure on a nerve or the spinal cord. Many spine specialists will perform surgery for severe neck pain associated with functional impairment due to one or two degenerated discs. But other surgeons feel there is not enough scientific evidence to warrant surgery for severe neck pain without arm pain or neurological changes.

The most common cause of severe neck pain is a damaged disc, and it can be seen on a high-quality MRI scan. If the pain location and intensity are consistent with the one or two bad discs on an MRI scan, surgery may help. However, when more than two discs are involved, the surgical success rate is much lower.

In order to resolve the question of whether surgery can help neck pain when there is no nerve compression, we performed a scientific study of the results of cervical fusion for neck pain, and our findings were published in a major scientific journal, *Spine*, in 1999. We continued to follow thirty-eight patients for a period of more than two years. We found that 79 percent of our patients improved significantly, and most were able to resume normal levels of activity. However, only a small number had complete relief of their pain. We continue to recommend surgery for our patients who have severe pain, poor function, and have not improved with medications, injections, and physical therapy.

If the specialist you see tells you that surgery is necessary to correct your problem, you might ask the surgeon for the names of some patients who have had similar surgeries (obviously, the specialist will need the patient's permission first). Choose a surgeon who does at least several spine surgeries each week. Make sure the surgeon will continue to provide care for you in the future, even if you do not get better. Do not feel shy or embarrassed about asking these questions. A physician should anticipate and welcome such questions, and be happy to make you as comfortable as possible about such a serious decision as surgery.

Types of Surgery

There are several different surgeries available to treat the cervical spine. The choice of surgery is determined by the diagnosis, the experience and philosophy of the surgeon, and a patient's overall medical condition.

When planning a neck surgery, the surgeon will decide whether to make the incision through the front of the neck (anterior) or through the back of the neck (posterior). The cervical discs and vertebrae are quite close to the skin in the front of the neck, which allows relatively easy access. The nerve canals can be opened, damaged or herniated discs removed, and pressure can be relieved from the spinal cord. Some of the advantages of operating through the front of the neck include: minimal loss of blood, a lower level of postoperative pain, ability to remove almost the entire disc, and low risk of damage to the spinal nerves and spinal cord. The most common complications are injury to a nerve that supplies the vocal cords and injury to the esophagus, but both are rare.

Posterior surgery is done far less often because it is more painful, has a longer recovery time, may have a higher incidence of nerve damage, and rarely relieves neck pain. However, an experienced surgeon can successfully remove a disc herniation compressing a nerve root or bone spurs compressing a nerve root or the spinal cord using this approach.

Whether to perform a fusion is another controversial aspect of anterior disc surgery. A fusion means that two or more vertebrae are joined, or fused together by adding bone to the space between them. During the healing process, the bone eventually knits solidly together and the spinal segments become one unit. There are few, if any, disadvantages to fusion. One fear is that fusion will lead to accelerated degeneration of the discs adjacent to the fused segments, but the scientific evidence suggests that this does not happen very often when all of the abnormal discs are included in the original fusion. On the other hand, there are several potential advantages to fusion. Stability is restored to the segment and it cannot deteriorate further and the normal cervical curve can be maintained, which helps protect the adjacent discs.

There is also some controversy about using donated bone from a bone bank because of the risk of infection. However, bone bank bone is very safe. In addition bone bank bone has been shown to work as well as a patient's own bone, and there will be no risk of pain from the site of the donated bone.

12
Treatment of Neck Pain: The Role of the Chiropractor

Chiropractic care is extremely popular, and in fact much of the primary care for neck pain is provided by chiropractors. Chiropractors are well trained to provide spinal manipulative therapy (SMT) for neck pain, and this form of treatment appears to help many people and to be generally safe. Modern chiropractors may combine SMT with training patients in exercise, body mechanics, and ergonomics. They may also offer massage, ultrasound, ice and heat treatments, and electrical stimulation. There is little or no controversy about these aspects of chiropractic treatment.

However, there are several philosophies of chiropractic, and, as a result, there may be significant disagreements among chiropractors themselves and between chiropractors and some medical doctors. On the other hand, there are enough areas of agreement between doctors of chiropractic and doctors of medicine that they should be able to work together to provide comprehensive care.

As a health care consumer, you should be informed about some of the differences between modern chiropractic thought and very traditional chiropractic. According to Samuel Homola, D.C., in his book *Inside Chiropractic*, even today chiropractors have different models of care. Many very traditional chiropractors still subscribe to the so-called "subluxation" theory, which maintains that nearly all illnesses stem from spinal misalignment and the resulting interruption of energy or nerve flow along the course of nerves that are in or arise from the spinal cord. Consequently, they may oppose vaccinations, antibiotic therapy for infectious diseases, and other medical treatments. In addition, they may embrace selling nutritional supplements, herbs, or other "natural" and unproven products. It is these chiropractors who have created much of the ill will between medical doctors and chiropractors. It does not make physiological sense that all diseases can have one cause—a problem with spinal alignment—nor that all diseases can have one treatment—spinal manipulation. However, most chiropractors who use SMT to treat neck and back problems are quite reputable and help many patients.

A panel of chiropractors and medical doctors recently evaluated the role of SMT for neck problems by reviewing the published research and combining their findings with their own clinical experiences. In his chapter in the recent chiropractic textbook *Conservative Management of Cervical Spine Syndromes*, an academic chiropractor, Dr. Kim Humphreys, presents another review of the scientific evidence regarding SMT. Both the expert panel and Dr. Humphreys agree that there is good evidence that SMT can provide short-term relief for many people with neck pain and that it is quite safe. However, neither source found any evidence showing benefits for long-term or preventative manipulation, which some chiropractors advocate. Although there are differences of opinion, many chiropractors feel children should not undergo SMT, and some question the value of preventative chiropractic care.

Spinal Manipulative Therapy (SMT)

The major emphasis of chiropractic care is spinal manipulative therapy (SMT), the best term to describe the types of therapies chiropractors use most often. There are two types of SMT, mobilization and manipulation. They differ in terms of the amplitude and speed of joint movement, and the patient's ability to remain in control of the movement. In mobilization, the chiropractor or other manual therapist applies gentle, rapid back-and-forth movements of differing amplitudes at a rate two to three cycles per second to a joint. There are no sudden thrusts, and the patient is still able to control the motion. The range of motion is extended gradually to relieve restriction and stiffness. In manipulation, the chiropractor typically applies a rapid, low-amplitude thrust that stretches a joint beyond its restricted range of motion, but not beyond its normal anatomic range. The patient is not in control of the degree of movement.

Effectiveness of Spinal Manipulative Therapy (SMT)

Acute Neck Pain

In acute neck pain, SMT can be helpful, although scientific studies report mixed results. Keep in mind that most people with acute neck pain will get better with or without treatment, so it is hard to know from the research that has been conducted whether the SMT helped or if the person would have gotten better anyway. That said, it appears that patients treated with SMT during the first few days of an episode of neck pain feel better one week later than patients treated only with medications. However, from the results of several studies, it is unlikely that SMT will change the way patients will feel six or twelve weeks later. In some research studies, patients who received SMT were slightly better two or three months later than those who just received a cervical collar and general advice about neck pain from their general medical physicians.

The consensus of experts appears to be that chiropractic helps some patients with acute neck pain feel better sooner, but probably does not significantly change the long-term outcome. If you are inclined to try chiropractic care, or have experienced relief in the past after treatment from a chiropractor, SMT is an appropriate treatment for three to four weeks. Then, if your neck pain improves, it may be appropriate to continue SMT for an additional four to six weeks while you begin strength and body mechanics training.

CHRONIC NECK PAIN

There are many causes for chronic neck pain, and unfortunately there are no studies that evaluate the effectiveness of SMT for each specific condition. When all patients with chronic neck pain are grouped together, some conclusions can be reached. There is good evidence that most patients treated with either SMT, aggressive strengthening, or physical therapy all get somewhat better with no differences in outcomes between these treatments. However, because there were no "placebo groups" in the studies, it is impossible to say whether the improvements were due to the passage of time and natural healing or to the specific effects of the treatment.

In one study that compared SMT to standard physical therapy and placebo (an inactive treatment), both SMT and standard physical therapy were equal in terms of effectiveness. Both treatments were better than a single visit to a general medical doctor, but neither was better than placebo. Almost all patients improved, which implies that it is the nonspecific effects of the treatment (placebo effect, see chapter 14) that helped rather than the treatment itself. There is some evidence that SMT provides short-term relief for patients with chronic neck pain, but less evidence that it produces any long-term relief.

SMT has both positives and negatives. If you are able to get relief that lasts several days and then use that period of improvement to exercise, SMT can be a very valuable addition to exercise and the practice of good body mechanics. In fact, there are patients who need one or two chiropractic treatments per month to keep their pain at a lower level and to maintain high function, and this is very reasonable treatment. There are downsides, however. Some patients become very dependent on manual treatment, and do not take responsibility for getting better. They may feel that they improve only when something is done *to* them, which may reinforce feelings of dependence and helplessness. There is also the concern that SMT over a period of years may result in excess joint laxity, which can create a new painful condition.

Frequency and Duration of SMT

There are no well established guidelines to suggest the optimum frequency and duration of SMT. During my research for this book, I interviewed several chiropractors. The consensus from these interviews was that it is appropriate to treat acute neck pain with SMT two to three times per week for three weeks. If the patient is not getting any meaningful improvement, then SMT should be discontinued. If the patient experiences significant improvement, but still has some pain, it is reasonable to continue treatments for an additional two to three sessions per week for three more weeks to a maximum of twelve to eighteen total sessions.

However, after this time period, the emphasis of chiropractic care should shift from reliance on SMT to training in body mechanics and strengthening the spine safely. There may be the need for occasional SMT as you begin training and for flares, but it should become only a small part of long-term and comprehensive treatment, not the major part. Very rarely do patients need long-term SMT. On the other hand, some people do quite well with one or two manual therapy sessions per month for flares or long-term symptom control. Many chiropractors themselves design and implement training programs for their patients, but others refer their patients to physical therapists.

Complications of SMT

One reason that medical doctors hesitate to recommend chiropractors for their own patients with neck pain is the fear of complications from SMT, but in fact complications are rare. One recent review found that only 110 cases of significant complications after cervical spine manipulation had been reported in the entire scientific literature. From this low incidence, the authors estimated that the incidence of significant complications may be as low as one for every 1 million to 2 million cervical manipulations.

The most feared complication is a stroke caused by compression of the arteries that run in the back part of the neck, but this is also a very rare event. There are no specific warning signs that might predict which patients are at risk for stroke following SMT. In general, though, chiropractors should not perform rotational manipulations in people with dizziness, light-headedness, very severe and/or acute headaches, or in people with prior strokes or diseases of other arteries. Practitioners should also use caution in patients with high blood pressure, heavy smokers, and the elderly. Injury to the spinal cord or a major nerve is very rare. Make sure that if you have any of the symptoms or illnesses mentioned above that you tell your chiropractor before any treatment begins.

Most complications are due to performing SMT on patients who are not interviewed carefully to detect any serious medical illness that may be present. People with infections, cancer, or benign tumors of the spine, or a history of bleeding problems, should not have SMT because they are more susceptible to serious complications.

Side effects are common after manipulation. The most common is a temporary increase in pain. You might also experience headaches and fatigue. If this happens, neck first aid (see chapter 7) might help. Before you leave the chiropractor's office, ask what to do if side effects occur.

OTHER TYPES OF MANUAL THERAPY

Massage Therapy

Massage is manual therapy directed toward the muscles and underlying soft tissues such as ligaments and tendons. Massage therapy can temporarily help because many people with neck pain have some degree of secondary muscle spasm that increases the pain from deeper structures. Massage can relieve some of the muscle spasm, but if there is no attention paid to the underlying cause, the spasm and muscle pain will recur.

Because it involves a "hands on" approach, massage can be soothing, relaxing, and "healing." It is important to remember that massage does not cure. However, any treatment that has low risk and provides some degree of pain relief is valuable. In addition, massage can be particularly helpful if it enables you to work harder in your strengthening program.

Massage also can provide psychological benefit. It is the laying on of hands in a supportive and nonjudgmental environment.

Rolfing

Rolfing is a form of deep tissue massage that purports to move the layers of fascia and improve mobility and local blood flow. Fascia are the connective tissues that surround the muscles and other body structures. "Rolfers," who follow the methods of the founder, Ida Rolf, Ph.D., believe that when fascia become too rigidly adherent, smooth motion is impaired and results in pain. The goal of the therapy is to realign abnormal soft tissues and restore normal soft-tissue mobility. During sixty- to ninety-minute sessions, Rolfers use their fingers, knuckles, and sometimes even their elbows or knees to apply deep pressure to all areas of the body. Rolfing can be painful. There is no evidence one way or the other of the value of Rolfing. Obviously, its practitioners and supporters strongly believe in its healing qualities.

Craniosacral Therapy

Craniosacral therapy is a treatment based on the belief that there are normal rhythm patterns or oscillations in the body tissues that come from the elasticity of soft tissues, gravity, and muscle contractions. Practitioners of craniosacral therapy say they can feel these rhythms by palpating the skull with their fingers or hands. They claim to feel the lines between the bones of the skull, and think they can tell if they are normal or not. They believe "abnormal rhythms" can be restored to normal, thus improving neck or low back pain and spinal balance.

To my knowledge, there is no documentation that these rhythms even exist, nor is there any evidence that craniosacral therapy is any more than a placebo. There are no reports of complications or damage due to this treatment, although some caution against using this method in infants or young children in whom the bones of the skull are not yet fully formed.

Reflexology

Reflexology is based on the theory that there are specific points on the feet that correspond to organ systems of the body. When there is illness or dysfunction of an internal organ, the corresponding points on the soles of the feet will be tender. Reflexology is not massage, but a system of applying pressure to the tender reflex points, thus hoping to improve the condition of the organ to which the point corresponds.

There is no scientific evidence to support or refute the technique for the treatment of pain. As with any alternative treatment, the risk may not be in the treatment itself, but in the failure to use medical treatments that could help, especially if there is a serious illness present.

DIET AND NUTRITIONAL SUPPLEMENTS

Some chiropractors sell nutritional programs and dietary supplements as part of their treatment of neck pain. Although it makes sense to achieve and maintain ideal body weight, especially to prevent and treat knee and hip problems, there is no scientific evidence that weight loss or nutritional programs have any effect on neck pain.

There are several best-selling books about the treatment of osteoarthritis with nutritional supplements, especially glucosamine and chondroitin (see chapter 14). However, the authors do not claim these supplements are effective for neck pain. In addition, they actually recommend a comprehensive plan using exercise, strengthening, weight loss, and relaxation training for joint pain. Although the nutritional supplements are just a small part of the program, they have received most of the attention.

Nutritional remedies offer no particular benefit and appear geared more to the financial health of the practitioner rather than the neck health of the patient.

13
Treatment of Neck Pain: The Role of the Physical Therapist

Physical therapists are health professionals who provide rehabilitation for a wide range of injuries and illnesses. They spend at least four years in college and then may spend additional time specializing. They help patients with strokes to regain function; patients with joint replacements to recover strength and mobility; and patients with heart attacks to recuperate with aerobic conditioning. Physical therapists (sometimes referred to simply as "PTs") also work with people who have sustained sports or industrial injuries to reduce their pain, increase function, prevent reinjury, and slow the progression of degenerative changes. Physical therapists help patients achieve independence and reinforce the ability to continue exercising without supervision. And since they are experts in the principles of body mechanics, physical therapists can instruct patients in the correct ways to move, thus helping to minimize patients' fears of reinjury. In addition, some physical therapists do ergonomic job site evaluations and recommend changes to improve working conditions. They are teachers, problem solvers, and health scientists—not technicians who just follow doctors' orders.

In the past, patients who had neck or low back pain were instructed to rest the injured body part until the pain decreased—essentially, to do nothing that hurt. This philosophy has changed as research showed that rest was not helpful after a few days, and early mobilization and return to activity after injury improved the speed of healing. However, it is important that people exercise in a safe manner to minimize the chances of reinjury. Physical therapists can facilitate the process of a safe return to activity. In modern physical therapy, patients actively participate in their own care and rehabilitation, and the therapist imparts the necessary skills to the patient to carry out the program.

In an older model of physical therapy, patients were passive recipients of treatments such as massage, spinal manipulative therapy (see chapter 12), diathermy (heat), or electrical stimulation of muscles. We now sometimes refer to this form of treatment disparagingly as "shake, bake, and ultraviolate" to suggest that it is not very useful and may be a waste of money and time. It is clear that such treatments do little more than maintain the status quo—that is, while they may make someone feel better temporarily, they do not address the underlying cause of pain or provide a way to become active again.

In some states, physical therapists can work independently of physicians, but other states require a doctor's prescription. This means that you must be referred by your doctor, and will not be able to go directly to a PT's office.

Why Is a Physical Therapist Necessary?

In the last two decades, physicians and other health professionals have accumulated a large amount of knowledge about neck pain, but most of that information has not been presented in a way that the general public could easily understand. Doctors are ultimately responsible for educating their patients about neck pain. However, they often refer their patients to physical therapists for this essential education, in part because doctors may not have the time to spend educating each individual patient.

In addition to teaching patients about their own anatomy and causes of neck pain, physical therapists set up and then supervise proper strength and body mechanics training programs. This expertise becomes a vital part of the recovery process.

For some readers, this book will provide much of the information that was available previously only from the doctors and therapists, although it is not meant to be a substitute for doctors or therapists. It is meant to make their work easier, because working with informed patients improves treatment success. In addition, after reading this book, many people will still benefit from professional help and advice, especially those who have pain or unanswered questions.

The program in this book can neither cover every situation nor help every person with neck pain—no book can. If you do not get better even after following the program in this book, you may respond to a professionally directed regime that is individualized for your needs. A good physical therapist can provide that direction, perhaps by identifying weaknesses in muscles that are not usually a problem or by observing nuances in the way you move, sit, stand, or exercise that contribute to your pain. Then the therapist can tailor a program to help correct bad habits and improper body mechanics. He or she will often demonstrate corrective and strengthening exercises in the office visit and assign exercises that you can do at home or in a gym. A therapist can also slow or increase the rate of progression of exercises to better suit your individual needs.

The physical therapist will also know when your treatment is not working, and further evaluation is needed. Then, the therapist can facilitate communication with your doctor.

PHYSICAL THERAPY EVALUATION

At your first visit, you can expect the physical therapist to conduct an independent assessment of your overall strength, flexibility, posture, body mechanics, and function. If you have neck pain, the PT will emphasize your cervical spine. Since neck posture and mechanics start with the low back, the therapist may also evaluate your lumbar spine, shoulders, and other muscles, bones, and joints.

Evaluation of Muscle Strength

It is important for the PT to ascertain the strength of the muscles in the front and back of your neck, as well as those of your upper back. There are several ways to do this. The PT may test your isometric muscle strength (see chapter 8) by measuring how long you can hold a muscle in its exercise position against gravity alone or with the additional resistance of a light weight. For isotonic testing, the therapist can count the number of repetitions of a certain exercise that you are able to complete with or without weights. There are also specialized strength-testing machines, but these are not practical for routine use. The machines do a good job, but they are expensive and the test results are not easily transferred to your gym or home exercise program. They increase rather than decrease your reliance on the therapist, and may slow your progress to an independent program.

Evaluation of Body Mechanics

No objective measures of body mechanics currently exist, so the PT will evaluate your body mechanics based on his or her expert impressions. In order to bring some consistency to the evaluation of body mechanics, we developed a series of functional tests to quantify each patient's body mechanics. These tests involve asking the patient to demonstrate important common postures or movements, which are:

- Rising from sitting on a chair to standing
- Changing from sitting on a chair to lying
- Sitting in neutral
- Reaching in front and overhead
- Bending at the waist

The therapist grades each posture or movement, and the final score provides an indication of the person's overall body mechanics. After the patient has been taught proper posture and body mechanics, the test can be repeated to monitor changes. Over time, there should be improvement in functional testing, which will carry over to activities of daily life.

Functional Capacity and Work Capacity Evaluations

Most people with neck problems are either working, planning to return to work, or attending school. As discussed in chapter 9, ergonomic factors (such as the layout and design of a work space) often determine whether a person can work safely. Of course, the worker's own physical capacities also influence his or her ability to do the job safely. A physical therapist can evaluate both of these important elements.

The purpose of a functional capacity evaluation (FCE) is to measure a person's tolerance for physical tasks such as lifting, carrying, bending, reaching, twisting, pushing, pulling, and sitting. An FCE also may identify deficits in body mechanics and strength that are necessary to perform these tasks safely, thus indicating targets for further treatment. The FCE can tell a treating doctor or an insurance company whether, when, or if a person is ready to return to work. To monitor progress, the FCE can be repeated several weeks or months later, usually in an abbreviated form.

A work capacity evaluation (WCE) includes the same types of measurements, but then compares the results with the physical demands of a particular job to see if the person is capable of performing that job safely. The WCE will indicate whether, when, or if a person can return to a specific job.

PHYSICAL THERAPY EDUCATION AND TRAINING

After evaluation, the next step the PT uses is educating you about good body mechanics and instructing you in correct ways to get stronger.

Strength Training

One of the most important things a physical therapist does is teach a person to strengthen muscles in a "spine-safe" manner. If you do these exercises properly, you can make significant gains in strength with little or no increase in pain. In chapter 8, I presented the most important exercises for the neck. However, not everyone can learn to exercise by reading a book and looking at drawings. Some people need the individual attention of a physical therapist or trainer (see page 207).

In addition, not every exercise is right for every person. For some people, one particular exercise will cause the pain to get worse, despite perfect technique. The therapist can observe you performing your exercises, analyze the way you do them, and, when necessary, substitute a different exercise to strengthen the same group of muscles.

Some patients make rapid progress in their strength training and soon are ready to go to a gym and use free weights or resistance equipment. Some of these machines can be quite challenging to the person with neck pain. Many therapists have gyms in their offices and can teach their patients to use them safely and properly. Others will accompany their patients to their local gyms or health clubs to help them learn proper technique, or refer their patients to a specially trained exercise trainer.

Body Mechanics Training

Another equally important role of a physical therapist is to teach patients how to use their bodies correctly. There are specific postures and movement patterns that apply to almost everyone (see chapter 9), but some individuals do some very specific and perhaps unusual tasks or activities. A physical therapist can evaluate these tasks to find ways for them to be done safely without risk of reinjury.

Some people can figure out safe ways of moving on their own, once they understand the basics of posture and movement. Others need the professional help of a therapist. This should not make someone feel inadequate. I tell my patients that it is much harder to learn to dance from a book than from a dance teacher!

Besides directing training in an office setting, a physical therapist may visit your job site or even go running, bicycling, or golfing with you to observe your mechanics and make improvements on the spot that can then be reinforced at future office visits.

Trainers and Physical Therapy Assistants

Some people need one-on-one treatment with a physical therapist. However, most of the basic exercises and body mechanics can be readily taught to a group of patients at the same time. You may benefit from group physical therapy, since you can also learn from observing other patients, and the group members often give each other encouragement. Group therapy is more efficient and more cost-effective, but less personal.

In addition, you can receive training from a certified athletic trainer or physical therapy assistant who is under the supervision and direction of a licensed physical therapist. After the PT designs the program, the trainer implements it. In this situation, you would still see your PT regularly for reevaluation. He or she will help solve problems, and modify the program as necessary. Trainers and physical therapy assistants are also an efficient use of resources.

14
Treatment of Neck Pain: Alternative and Complementary Therapies

More people are turning toward alternative health care for the treatment of pain. Some are disenchanted with the health care system, and have lost faith in doctors and pharmaceutical companies. Others want to try treatments that appear natural and organic, not synthetic or chemical. As a result, alternative health care practitioners have flourished.

A study published in January 1993 in the prestigious *New England Journal of Medicine* stated that as many as one in three Americans used some form of unconventional health care, but the authors included relaxation training and chiropractic as alternatives in their survey. They also stated that the public made more visits to and spent more money on alternative health care providers than primary care physicians. This, too, may be a bit misleading because the authors included massage as alternative health care, even if the patients had no medical illnesses. But even though the numbers are not that high, it is clear that the public is taking advantage of alternative and complementary health pratices.

Many practitioners of alternative or complementary health care techniques and manufacturers of dietary supplements make claims that their treatments have succeeded where traditional medical care has failed. However, alternative health care practitioners do not need to prove their claims because they are not held to the same high scientific standards as medical doctors by government agencies, licensing boards, or their peers.

To make matters even more difficult, there are no definitions of complementary, unconventional, or alternative medicine that everyone can agree upon. Margaret Angell and Jerome Kasirer, editors of the *New England Journal of Medicine*, feel that what distinguishes alternative medicine from conventional medicine is that alternative treatments have not been scientifically tested for efficacy or safety. Furthermore, advocates of alternative medicine deny the need for such testing and depend instead on anecdotes and theories. They may claim that their treatments are not testable by scientific methods. Angell and Kasirer feel many of the ideologies of alternative medicine ignore biologic mechanisms, disparage modern science, and rely on practices based on ancient remedies, which they see as more potent and less toxic. Some alternative practitioners feel that just because some of these treatments have survived for hundreds or thousands of years, they must work or they would have disappeared.

Another definition of alternative medicine, paraphrased from articles by Tim Gorski, M.D., Associate Editor, *Scientific Review of Alternative Medicine* and David Eisenberg, M.D., Beth Israel Hospital, Boston, Massachusetts, is "health care practices that are not in conformity with the standards of the medical community. In turn, standards of the medical community are methods that have been proven to be truly effective by rigorous scientific standards. Complementary medicine practices are those that add to or complement medical practices and quality of life."

WHY PEOPLE GET BETTER

People get better for many reasons, including the cyclical nature of the pain or illness, the specific effects of treatment (such as antibiotics given to treat an infection), and the nonspecific effects of treatment (such as the placebo effect discussed on page 211). Each of these possibilities must be considered when evaluating traditional medical treatments and when judging alternative or complementary therapies. Although some alternatives have been proven effective, most are shown to be ineffective when subjected to the same rigorous scientific evaluations required of medical treatments. Often, claims of success are based on patient testimonials, a type of advertising, not science. Manufacturers of dietary supplements know that compelling anecdotes will go a long way toward selling their products, and use testimonials to great advantage. Fortunately, researchers and government agencies finally are evaluating the safety and effectiveness of some popular alternative health care treatments.

Many medical problems such as neck pain are cyclical. There are times when pain is better and times when it is worse. The implication of the cyclical nature of pain is that most exacerbations of pain will improve on their own with or without treatment. But patients tend to go to their health care providers when pain is worse. They receive treatment, and because they soon feel better, both the patient and the health care provider might assume falsely that the improvement is due to the treatment rather than the cyclical nature of the problem. If this pattern is repeated often enough, it reinforces the mistaken belief that the treatment was responsible for the improvement rather than the natural ebbs and flows of the pain or illness.

Another reason people get better is the nonspecific effect of treatment, better known as the placebo effect. The placebo effect is the nonspecific result of treatment. When there is a placebo response, the treatment worked because it triggered the body's own inner resources, not because the treatment had specific healing benefits. A placebo effect does not mean the pain is psychological ("all in your head") or that it is not real. A placebo can relieve the pain of wisdom tooth extraction. A placebo response just means the improvement was due to the patient's own internal pain-fighting mechanisms, which were triggered by treatment. It is the act of being treated, not the treatment itself that helps. Nonspecific factors that may trigger the placebo effect include patients' expectations, cultural beliefs, the concern and attention of the health care provider, and the setting of the treatment. Scientists must account for the placebo effect in their research, but most alternative health care providers do not. The fact that the patient got better should not be used as "proof" that any remedy, traditional or alternative, works.

Specific effects of treatment are benefits that are directly due to the content and activity of the treatment. For example, penicillin is a specific treatment for some types of pneumonia. Morphine is an effective treatment for severe pain. Medical doctors must prove that their treatments work because of the specific activity of the treatment, not the nonspecific effects of just being treated. In order to test a treatment, researchers will give some patients placebo treatment and others the treatment that is being tested. Only if the active treatment yields significantly better results than the placebo will researchers know the treatment is truly effective.

Why Unproven Remedies Are So Popular

There are many explanations for the popularity of alternative therapies. One is the failure to differentiate between correlation and causation. Events that occur sequentially can be correlated or associated without there being the direct link of cause and effect. For instance, many people think that cold weather causes colds, but this is not the case. Colds are due to viruses. Although there is an increased incidence of colds during periods of cold weather (correlation), the real reason (causation) for the increased incidence of colds is that people gather together indoors where there is poor ventilation and a greater opportunity for transmission of the viruses that cause the colds.

ARE ALTERNATIVE REMEDIES DANGEROUS?

Two of the potential dangers of alternative or complementary medicine are the failure to recognize serious medical illnesses that require conventional medical treatment and the danger of the alternative therapies themselves. Fortunately, most people use alternative therapies for health maintenance or for minor problems. There are reported cases, however, of people who became ill after taking herbal remedies that contained dangerously high concentrations of digitalis or estrogens. Recently, there have been reports that the herbal therapy Saint-John's-Wort, used for depression, negatively interacts with some important conventional medications, rendering them toxic or ineffective. This is an exception, because for the most part, herbal or homeopathic remedies are safe.

A REVIEW OF SOME ALTERNATIVE THERAPIES

Acupuncture

Acupuncture is a healing art that has been practiced for more than two thousand years. It was originally developed in China, but its use has spread throughout the world. It continues to be popular for the treatment of pain. Although there are several types of acupuncture, most depend on using very thin needles of varying lengths to stimulate specific points on the skin that correlate with so-called channels of energy flows. Traditional acupuncture is practiced according to the principles of Chinese medicine that theorize most illnesses are due to imbalance in the body's energy flows. Acupuncture attempts to restore the energy balance by placing needles along points that represent the paths of these energy flows, called meridians. Less traditional acupuncturists place needles into tender points, not just meridian lines. Others use electrical rather than manual stimulation of needles.

Acupuncture may work to reduce pain in some people. Medical science has not learned all of the ways acupuncture works, but several mechanisms have been proposed. Acupuncture may stimulate the release of endorphins, the body's own pain-fighting hormones. It also stimulates nerves other than the ones carrying the message of pain, and thereby may partially block the transmission of the pain signal to the brain (see chapter 2).

Interestingly, acupuncture has only been shown to be helpful in problems such as pain or nausea that are subjective and not directly measurable. There are no studies to show acupuncture is useful for conditions that are measurable by objective tests, such as liver, kidney, or heart disease. Many scientific studies have looked at the effectiveness of acupuncture for low back pain, and the results are mixed. Some studies have found acupuncture helpful, but others have not. One writer in a leading scientific journal stated that the better the quality of the study, the less the likelihood to be able to show any benefit from acupuncture. There is no information about the value of acupuncture for neck pain. There is sufficient scientific data to say that acupuncture is effective for dental pain, and some suggestions that acupuncture helps some patients with menstrual cramps, tennis elbow, and fibromyalgia.

Acupuncture has few side effects, and if sterile or disposable needles are used, it is safe. Therefore, it may be worth trying acupuncture for three to six weeks. If you do not experience any significant or sustained benefit, then the acupuncture is not working. If there is meaningful improvement, acupuncture can be continued. Acupuncturists should be certified, and in some states licensed. Some resources to find a certified acupuncturist are listed in appendix B.

Meditation

Meditation is also an ancient technique. The goal during meditation is to free the mind from intrusive thoughts. Eventually, meditation is purported to provide peace of mind, body, and spirit. Although it is still used for spiritual purposes today, meditation has also become popular as a relaxation technique to manage stress, pain, and high blood pressure (see chapter 17). There are many types of meditation, and all seem to provide similar benefits of relaxation and stress reduction. In most techniques, there is intense focus on some single thing—breath, candlelight, a sound, or footsteps. By staying focused, the mind is quieted. Eventually, the peace of mind becomes natural and lasts beyond the period of meditation.

Meditation requires work and must be practiced on a regular basis to be beneficial. It is much more difficult than it seems. Those new to the discipline may find they have a tendency to fall asleep or to daydream. Thoughts intrude constantly. As a result, many people do better learning to meditate with a teacher and in a group. Often meditation practice is combined with an exploration of spiritual beliefs. If practiced diligently, meditation may provide relief from some of the pain related to stress and anxiety.

Magnets

The use of magnets to treat muscle and joint pain has become popular lately. They are being marketed in catalogs, health food stores, chiropractors' offices, and even dry cleaning shops. Magnets can be purchased to put under a pillow, on top of a mattress, in shoes, or to be wrapped around the back, knees, or other joints. One firm that sells magnets for pain relief has increased its sales from $3 million in 1989 to $150 million in 1998!

Manufacturers offer many seemingly attractive theories about why magnets work, none of which make physical or biological sense. Some state magnets can improve blood flow, nerve function, and oxygenation of vital tissues, as well as decrease deposits on the walls of blood vessels. Others say the earth's magnetic field has decreased, which may be a cause of "magnetic field deficiency syndrome." Skeptics argue that the magnets used for pain relief could not penetrate into the body more than one or two millimeters and have never been shown to do anything to major biological systems.

A recent study of the use of magnets for the treatment of low back pain showed no benefits, and there are no studies about the use of magnets for the treatment of neck pain. However, there is one well-performed scientific study of patients with pain due to the late effects of polio. Patients who were treated with active magnetized magnets had greater pain reduction than those treated with demagnetized magnets. These were short-term results only, and there are no long-term data. Nevertheless, these results must make us consider the possibility that magnet therapy can help some people. It is very premature to apply this small study to every person with pain.

Magnets are safe. Some can be very expensive, but most are not. The benefits are probably due to the placebo effect, but given the low risk, they may be worth trying.

Diet and Nutritional Supplements

There are many health claims for various dietary treatments of pain. As might be expected, most are based more on testimonials than science. There is no doubt that a healthy diet is good for everyone, but there is no evidence that any particular diet or nutritional supplements will help pain.

It is abundantly clear that obesity is unhealthy and carrying excess body weight is particularly bad for the knees and hips. There may be an increased incidence of low back pain in people who are severely overweight as well. Hip and knee pain may improve with weight reduction because the joints will have less load to bear, but there is no evidence that weight loss helps low back pain or neck pain. It may be the ratio of fat to muscle that is more important than the actual body weight. If the muscles are strong enough to carry it, some excess weight may not be important. Put another way, "It's not what you weigh, it's what it's made of."

Excess weight in the chest or abdomen may tend to pull the upper part of the body forward, which will pull the head and neck forward as well. This puts excessive strain on neck muscles, discs, and joints. Treatment would combine weight loss with strengthening the muscles of the upper back.

Dietary Supplements

GLUCOSAMINE AND CHONDROITIN

Glucosamine and chondroitin are dietary supplements that have become extremely popular for the treatment of arthritis since the books *The Arthritis Cure* and *Maximizing the Arthritis Cure*, by Dr. Jason Theodosakis, M.D., Brenda Adderly, M.H.A., and Barry Fox, Ph.D., were published. It is theorized that glucosamine stimulates the production of specialized proteins in joints, and this in turn slows the breakdown of cartilage and thereby slows the progression of arthritis. Glucosamine may have some anti-inflammatory properties as well. Some patients have reported decreased joint pain, decreased swelling, and improved joint function after using glucosamine. Adding chondroitin theoretically slows the breakdown of cartilage even more and adds to the benefits of glucosamine.

Proponents of glucosamine and chondroitin refer to scientific studies to support their theories. Unfortunately, most of these studies were poorly designed and their conclusions may not be justified by the data. There are no studies to document long-term benefit or long-term safety, and these supplements are not regulated by the FDA since they are not considered drugs. High-quality studies have been started that will critically evaluate the role of these supplements for joint pain.

However, there is some research that clarifies the role of these two supplements. Two studies, one concerning Navy SEALs and another patients from Canada, showed that glucosamine and chondroitin taken together relieved knee pain more than a placebo, and both studies found the combination to be safe. The results were only short-term, and there has not been long-term follow-up of either group. In a recent study from Belgium, patients who took glucosamine had less knee pain and perhaps less joint space narrowing on X-rays than patients on placebo. This, too, is encouraging research.

Unfortunately, there are no studies of the value of glucosamine or chondroitin for the treatment of either neck or low back pain. The cartilage of the discs of the spine share some of the same elements as the knees, but discs have a very poor blood supply, which might limit the effectiveness of the supplements. Even the major proponents of glucosamine and chondroitin, Dr. Theodosakis, M.D., University of Arizona College of Medicine, and his associates do not feel these treatments are effective for disc problems, perhaps because discs do not have very effective self-repair mechanisms. However, since facet joint problems cause neck pain in a substantial number of people, these supplements may be useful in these instances.

MSM (METHYLSULFONYLMETHANE)

MSM is a nutritional supplement that has been proposed as yet another miracle treatment for osteoarthritis, rheumatoid arthritis, low back pain, bladder pain, and other medical conditions. In the book *The Miracle of MSM: The Natural Solution for Pain*, by Stanley W. Jacob, M.D., Ronald M. Lawrence, M.D., Ph.D., and Martin Zucker, the authors claim great success for their product when it is used to treat these and other medical illnesses. Their optimism is based on personal experiences, but there are no good scientific studies to prove the value of MSM. On the other hand, there are no studies to show it does not work, and MSM does not appear to be associated with significant risk.

SHARK CARTILAGE

Shark cartilage is another dietary supplement publicized as a treatment for both arthritis and cancer. A 1992 book entitled *Sharks Don't Get Cancer* by William Lane and Linda Comac, contributed greatly to the popularity of this supplement, which can cost as much as $700 for a month's supply. There is no evidence that shark cartilage helps either cancer, reverses osteoporosis, or helps joint pain.

Therapeutic Touch

Therapeutic touch is a technique that allegedly manipulates the energy field that its proponents believe surrounds each patient. Although practitioners do not actually put their hands on the patient, they claim that they can help people by balancing the fields of energy that emanate from their bodies. However, when scientists performed an experiment to determine if an experienced practitioner of therapeutic touch could feel an energy field, she could not. Other scientists looked at all of the published research on therapeutic touch. Despite great claims made by its practitioners, there is no evidence to show it works. All of the successes noted were anecdotal and no better than that which would be expected from a placebo treatment.

15
Sports and Other Recreational Activities

It may seem paradoxical that athletics can be a cause of neck pain, and that exercise is a major part of the solution. In this chapter, I discuss the ergonomic challenges of some of the sports people enjoy most—bicycling, running, tennis, swimming, and golf. I also discuss some popular recreational activities—gardening, reading, and watching movies and television. Your neck pain does not have to prevent your participation in these activities, provided you use proper body mechanics. This chapter does not include a discussion about contact sports or major team sports such as football or basketball.

SPORTS

Using good body mechanics is fundamental to enjoying sports and other recreational activities. In any sport, athletes with excellent technique and mechanics perform better than those with mediocre technique. Correspondingly, people with neck pain who are able to use good mechanics can participate without feeling worse, but those with poor technique will hurt and probably have to stop. With some modifications particularized to each activity, the same principles of ergonomics outlined in chapter 9 can be applied to bicycling, golf, tennis, running, swimming, and other sports.

Bicycling

Some of the causes of neck pain in bicyclists are poor head position (too much extension or flexion); road vibration; and strain and fatigue of the muscles in the back of the neck, shoulders, and between the shoulder blades—the muscles that support the head and upper body while riding. Most of these problems can be overcome because they are the result of poor cycling posture and technique or a bicycle that is not adjusted properly.

Riding Posture and Technique

Bicycling is a complex variation of sitting. To achieve good riding form and posture, you should follow the same guidelines as those outlined in chapter 9 for good sitting posture. Although it is nearly impossible to ride with perfect sitting posture, it is still important to maintain as much lumbar lordosis (an inward curve of your lower back) as possible to keep your chest and upper back upright, and to keep your head and neck in neutral position. Most of the forward leaning should occur at the hip joints (hip hinge, see chapter 9), not in the low back. If you lose your lumbar lordosis, your upper back will become too rounded and horizontal, which will force you to "crane" your neck into excess extension so you can see the road ahead. In addition, if your helmet rides too low on your head or your visor extends too far forward, the problem of overextension will be accentuated even more. Excess extension places strain on the facet joints.

If you ride with poor posture, especially if you are riding with poor lumbar lordosis, your head may stick out in front of your body. Gravity pulls your head down into flexion, and because your head is too far in front of your chest, there is no support from its base, the upper back. To fight the tendency for your head to sag or droop, the muscles of the back of your neck must work quite hard, and if they are not strong enough, they will be strained and become painful. Of course, the treatment is to ride with better posture and to strengthen these important but often overlooked riding muscles (see chapter 8).

A good way to learn to ride with proper sitting posture with the best possible lumbar lordosis is to use adhesive tape as a teaching tool. While you are standing, have a friend put a two- or three-inch-wide strip of adhesive tape up the middle of your spine from the tip of your tailbone to the bottom of your shoulder blades. Then, when you lose the lordosis while you are sitting on your bicycle saddle, the tape will pull and signal you that your back has sagged. Soon you will develop the feel of proper form. You can extend the tape higher, to the base of your skull, if you shave your neck. Then the tape will let you know when your head and neck sag.

It is also good to change your position frequently during a ride. You can periodically pedal standing up, especially during long rides or when ascending hills. Although standing on your pedals causes you to lose some efficiency, this loss is balanced by the decreased strain on the neck and other body parts.

Your arms bear a significant amount of your upper body weight while riding. If your posture is too rigid, more vibration than necessary will be transmitted to your shoulders and neck. It is important to ride with your elbows loose and unlocked and to change the position of your hands frequently. Road or touring bike riders should spend as little time as possible holding on to the lower part of the handlebars (the drops).

BICYCLE ADJUSTMENT

The major elements of bicycle design (called bicycle geometry by avid cyclists) that affect the neck are the length of the tube that runs from the seat to the handlebars (top tube); the height, position, and type of handlebars; and the height of the saddle. The length of the top tube basically determines the length of the bicycle. If the top tube is too long, you must stretch to reach the handlebars, a posture that rounds both your lower and upper back and forces your neck into excess extension. A shorter top tube will help you to sit upright. Unfortunately, the length of the top tube cannot be changed, so it is important to check this feature before you purchase a bike. You can also shorten the effective length of the bicycle by moving the seat forward, or getting a new stem (the part that connects the handlebars to the frame) that is designed to bring the handlebars closer to the rider.

Handlebars that are too low also cause you to round your upper and lower back, again putting your neck into excess extension. You can raise the height of the handlebars so that you can sit upright. In addition, the type of handlebars usually found on mountain bikes is better for your neck than the "drop-type" handlebars supplied with road and touring bikes. Although the upright position will increase the air resistance slightly, the difference would not be noticed by the average recreational rider.

Shock absorbers on the front of your bike can be of some value, and are now available on moderately priced mountain bikes. Rear shocks may add even more damping of the surface bumps and vibrations. You can decrease some of these road bumps and vibrations by simply riding with your elbows loose and bent.

STRETCHES

When you are doing long rides, it is important to take frequent breaks to rest and stretch. During each break, drink water and do a few neutralization exercises, particularly chin retractions, neck extensions, and rotations (see chapter 7). It also feels good to stretch the muscles between your shoulder blades, the scapulae pinching exercise (figure 16). Place your palms together with your arms dangling down behind your butt. Gently squeeze your shoulder blades toward each other. Then lift your hands upward while keeping your elbows straight. You will feel a stretch between your shoulder blades, which neutralizes the sustained bent forward riding position.

Running

Surprisingly, running does not pose much of a threat to the neck if you run with a smooth stride and avoid bouncing. It is probably better to run on a soft surface such as a track than on city sidewalks. Good running shoes will help absorb some of the shock as well.

Tennis

The main challenges to the neck from tennis are the serve, overhead shots, and backhands. Tennis players may be prone to facet joint problems because they look up and rotate to one side frequently and rapidly, particularly when serving or hitting an overhead shot. The solution is to change your form for these shots by playing the ball more in front of you. At first, this will feel awkward and you might lose some power. But when you master the technique, your power will return. You may need a few lessons from a tennis pro who understands these concepts.

The problems with the backhand shot occur when you are "beaten," and the ball is somewhat behind you. Then there is a tendency to rotate your upper body and neck excessively to your backhand side, which can put excess torque on your neck. There is no good way to hit these balls, and it may be better to let them go than risk harming your neck.

Swimming

Swimming is an excellent sport for aerobic training and strengthening, and it has the advantage that your neck does not bear the weight of your head. The most popular strokes are the crawl, breaststroke, backstroke, and sidestroke, each of which is quite different in its effect on the neck. The crawl may cause excess neck rotation, the breaststroke excess extension, and the backstroke too much flexion.

When doing the crawl, most swimmers rotate their heads and necks to take a breath, which may cause neck strain. You can avoid excess neck rotation by turning your whole body like a log for each breath, but this requires advanced swimming skill. An alternative is to wear a mask and snorkel so you can keep your neck in good alignment.

It is very difficult to swim the breaststroke and avoid excess cervical extension unless you are an excellent swimmer and can elevate your entire upper body as a whole with each stroke. If you like doing the breaststroke, you might need coaching from an instructor to work on your stroke to avoid cervical extension. You will need very strong arms and pectoral muscles and an excellent technique to do the breaststroke if you have chronic neck pain.

Backstroke can provide excellent exercise and puts minimal strain on your neck. Many people doing the backstroke have a tendency to rotate their neck and head to avoid colliding with the end of the pool. This can be avoided by knowing the "landmarks" on the sides of the pool or the walls of the room to better gauge when you are nearing the edge of the pool. Your neck should be in a neutral position with just enough flexion at the base of the skull to keep your face out of the water.

An excellent way to get a good workout in the water is to use an Aqua-Jogger belt, which floats you vertically rather than horizontally. You can jog in place to strengthen your legs and abdomen, use the resistance of the water to strengthen your arms, and get a good aerobic workout as well. Although there are no specific neck exercises, it is an excellent way to stay in shape with minimal risk of a flare.

Golf

Golfers face problems when they are addressing the ball prior to hitting it, at the end of the backswing, and at the end of the follow-through. Some golfers stare at the ball for long periods, especially when putting. They stand almost frozen, bent at the waist, neck flexed, and eyes looking down, a posture that is not good for anyone, let alone a person with neck pain. It is preferable to stand slightly back from the ball with your knees bent slightly, and your head and neck near neutral. Although this position usually feels awkward at first, it will become natural with repetition. Standing to putt is an opportunity to use the neck hinge (figure 27), since it is not possible to look down at a golf ball and use perfect body mechanics.

During the backswing, your head initially is looking down at the ball, but your shoulders rotate during the backswing. This essentially turns your neck while it is flexed, a bad position for your neck. You must shorten your backswing to avoid excess rotation of your shoulders.

There are many complexities to the golf swing. Only an expert can fully analyze your swing to determine if there are problems with it that contribute to neck pain. An organization that specifically helps golfers with back and neck problems is Back to Golf. Their Web site is in appendix B.

OTHER RECREATIONAL ACTIVITIES

Reading

Holding your neck for long periods in a flexed position strains the discs and possibly the facet joints. Yet, this is the position that most people use while reading when you place the reading material in your lap or on a desk surface. The height of the reading material is too low and almost forces your posture to be bad. Reading in bed may also put your neck into flexion, especially when your head is held bent forward by a stack of pillows.

There is a solution for each of these problems. When you are reading in a chair, the back of the chair should be high enough to support your neck. In addition, your neck should be in neutral and you should hold your reading material in front of your eyes. To sustain this awkward position, you can place your elbows on the armrests of the chair or rest them on your rib cage. If you need to look down slightly, use the skull hinge technique (figure 27). Then it is a simple matter to bring the reading material up to eye level without stressing your neck. When reading at a desk, make sure it is at the proper height and angle or use a slant board (see chapter 9).

Reading in bed is difficult under any circumstances. One good way is to lie in the neck rest position (see chapter 7) and hold the reading material in your outstretched arms, but this is awkward and your arms will probably tire quickly. A better way is to use a large foam wedge that will support your head, neck, and upper back when you hold the reading material in front of your eyes as described above. These are generally available in large department stores, the Back Saver catalog, or Relax the Back Stores.

Gardening

Using tools while you are standing, and working with your hands in the soil, can both endanger your neck while you are gardening. To use tools such as shovels, rakes, or hoes, get them with handles long enough to allow you to stand up straight while using them. You should stand about three feet away from the area you are working so that you do not have to bend your head and neck forward to look at the ground. To rake, shovel, or hoe, rock your whole body forward and backward at your knees and ankles rather than bend repeatedly at the waist.

To work in the dirt with your hands or with a short-handled tool such as a trowel, it is particularly important to keep your neck neutral. It is best to kneel on your knees with a pad under them, rather than to stand and bend at the waist. Squatting works well for many gardeners.

At the Movies

Sitting too close to the screen will force your neck into extension. It is even worse if you are seated off to one side, because then there is extension plus rotation. Both of these positions are bad for the facet joints. The only solution is to get to the theater early so that you can sit farther back and in the middle section. If you slouch in your seat, you will lose your lumbar lordosis, which will push your head and neck into flexion.

Television

If you are going to watch television, have the screen at about eye level. Do not slouch down in a soft chair or couch because that will bring your head forward. If you watch television in bed, sit up straight against the headboard or buy a foam wedge as described on page 228.

16
The Psychology of Pain

The relationship between the mind and the body has been discussed and debated by physicians and philosophers for centuries. This relationship is especially complex with respect to pain because pain can cause psychological problems, and psychological illnesses can make pain worse. In our society, we readily accept physical problems, but some people feel that psychological problems signify weakness and should not be revealed. Yet, almost everybody with chronic pain has some psychological reaction, which, if overlooked by the doctor or denied by the patient, decreases the chances of successful treatment.

One of the best definitions of pain is the one used by the International Association for the Study of Pain (IASP). It begins with the words: "Pain is an unpleasant sensory and emotional experience. . . ." "Sensory" denotes the physical part of the pain, and "emotional" means the psychological part. In some people, the sensory (physical) component of pain is more prominent, while in others, especially some people with chronic pain, the emotional aspects may dominate. For most people with chronic pain, both play a role.

In every type of pain, signals originate at the site of the injury, travel up the spinal cord, and are finally processed in the brain, where they are experienced as pain. The signals travel at the speed of electricity, and therefore we feel the pain of an acute injury almost instantly. Whether pain is caused by a bad disc in the neck, a sprained ankle, or cancer, the brain is the final site and interpreter of the pain message. Obviously, emotions are also processed in the brain, so it should not be surprising that psychological factors play an important role in the overall perception of pain.

PSYCHOLOGICAL DISORDERS AND PAIN: CAUSE OR EFFECT?

Everyone involved with a person in pain—the doctor, the patient, and the patient's family—recognizes that psychological issues are a part of the pain experience. However, when we think about pain and psychological problems, we are faced with the classic problem of the chicken and the egg. Which came first, the pain or the psychological disorder? Did the pain cause the psychological problem or is the psychological disorder the cause of the pain? There is no answer to this riddle because both situations exist. Constant pain can cause psychological problems such as depression or anxiety; psychological problems can play an important role in making pain worse, and, rarely, psychological illness can be the sole cause of pain.

Doctors who specialize in pain have learned a great deal from two recent research studies. In one, a group of psychologists studied the psychological responses to neck pain caused by car accidents. They administered written and verbal psychological tests to patients within one week of their accidents, and then administered the same tests again three months and then twenty-four months later. Just after the injury, there were no differences in psychological test results between those patients who eventually recovered and those who did not! But by three months after the injury, 81 percent of the patients who were still in pain had begun to develop psychological changes, and these changes were still present two years later in 69 percent of the patients who still had pain. These results strongly suggest that psychological changes in patients with chronic neck pain due to car accidents are usually due to the pain, not the cause of it. It is also remarkable that regardless of the initial psychological condition of the accident victim, two years after the accident, one-third of these patients still had neck pain that was bad enough to interfere with their lives.

In another study, patients with neck pain due to facet joint injuries (see chapter 2), who had developed psychological problems, were treated by heating the nerves to the joints, a procedure called medial branch neurotomy (see chapter 3). This procedure effectively relieves pain that is coming from facet joints for a period of nine to eighteen months. The researchers noted that when the pain improved, the psychological problems also improved. However, when the pain recurred, the psychological problems recurred soon after. Then, when the neurotomy was done a second time and the pain improved again, the psychological problems also got better. These results strongly suggest that in many patients, the chronic pain is the cause of the psychological problems.

Pain Psychoneurology

There are two terms that are frequently confused by professionals and laypersons alike: pain threshold and pain tolerance. Pain threshold describes the point at which a person becomes aware that a stimulus is painful. The International Association for the Study of Pain (IASP) defines pain threshold as the least experience of pain that a person can recognize. Although it may seem surprising, pain threshold is roughly the same in everyone, at least in laboratory testing. When heat is applied to skin and the temperature is gradually raised, most people perceive the heat as being painful at about the same temperature—the pain threshold.

However, pain tolerance varies quite a bit from person to person and also in the same person at different times and under different circumstances. Pain tolerance is the amount of pain a person can stand or tolerate. IASP defines pain tolerance as the greatest level of pain that a person is prepared to tolerate. There are many variables that contribute to pain tolerance, and psychological factors are among the most important. In some people, a minor injury will cause a great deal of pain, but in another person the same injury will just be annoying. Professional athletes continue to play despite painful injuries, but other people with the same injuries would be off work and home in bed. How can this be?

Variations in pain tolerance are a fascinating aspect of human nature. Pain is not a sensation like vision or hearing. We are not "hardwired" for pain. Many factors modify pain signals as they travel from the site of injury to the brain—some serve to decrease the pain and others increase it. Our perception of pain is the sum of many factors that include heredity, culture, environment, childhood experiences, and, perhaps most important, psychological state.

ACUTE PAIN VERSUS CHRONIC PAIN

Everybody has had pain, usually from an injury or an accident. In most cases, as the injury healed, the pain improved and eventually went away. This type of pain is called acute pain. The cause of acute pain is usually known and includes things like a sprained ankle or a broken wrist. In acute pain, the nervous system reacts by signaling the body's endocrine system to release powerful hormonelike chemicals into the bloodstream. These hormones can raise the heart rate and blood pressure and speed up breathing. The injured person may sweat and get goose bumps. This is the famous "fight or flight" mechanism, so called because these reactions prepare the body to either do battle or run away. Acute pain serves as a warning that something is wrong. The most common psychological responses to acute pain are anxiety and fear.

Chronic pain is different. There is no exact time period over which acute pain becomes chronic. By definition, pain that persists well beyond the time it usually takes that type of injury to heal is considered chronic. Chronic pain hurts just as much as acute pain, but it is different in many ways. For example, the pain may not be localized, and may spread to other areas of the body that were not originally injured. The fight or flight response is replaced by many of the same symptoms seen in people with depression, such as problems with sleep, appetite, loss of sex drive, and low energy. Eventually, two problems may exist—pain and depression.

Pain Behavior

One of the problems with diagnosing and treating pain is that pain is invisible. Pain is an inner experience that is known only to the person who hurts. One person cannot feel or experience another person's pain, pain cannot be measured, and there are no objective tests for pain. Therefore, doctors must rely totally on what their patients tell them, although we use the examination and test results to try and explain the pain. However, the *effects* of pain are visible, because pain causes people to behave in ways that can be observed by others. The way people act when they hurt is called pain behavior. A man who bangs his elbow might rub it, a woman with appendicitis may hold her belly, an animal licks its wound—these are all pain behaviors. They are observable by others. Some pain behaviors are normal; some are abnormal. Some pain behaviors may help healing; others may make pain last longer and lead to impairment or disability.

Planned reactions to pain are called conscious behaviors, such as putting ice on a painful area. Unplanned reactions to pain are called unconscious pain behaviors. Examples include rubbing a sore neck or limping on a sore ankle. These types of pain behaviors are rarely a problem, and can even be useful. In acute pain, some behaviors seem "designed" by nature to help the injured person rest and encourage healing. Pain behaviors may keep someone from using an injured body part too soon. Rest increases the chances of healing and decreases the chances of reinjury. The first-aid advice "Keep off the injured part until the pain decreases" sums up the idea of appropriate pain behavior. When the injury heals and pain diminishes, the pain behavior no longer serves a useful function, and should disappear on its own.

However, there are types of pain behaviors that are more subtle, and potentially more harmful, because they bring certain social or psychological benefits to the person with pain. These rewards for pain may be so positive that they can cause a person to unconsciously continue to have pain. For instance, pain behaviors that allow a person to avoid unpleasant things such as a bad job or a nagging spouse may serve to reinforce the pain and keep it going. Pain behaviors that bring special attention, money, or sympathy that might not be available otherwise might also unconsciously prolong the pain.

Behaviors that are appropriate for the situation are considered normal, and those that are inappropriate for the situation are considered abnormal. Pain behaviors may be considered abnormal when the reactions appear out of proportion to the events or conditions. For instance, if a doctor gently touches a person with a sore neck and that person screams out in pain, this would be abnormal pain behavior. If a person with a sore neck stays in bed all day, this is most likely abnormal pain behavior. Interestingly, if a player with a broken leg tries to get back into a football game, this is also abnormal pain behavior, although some fans might think it is admirable.

If an injury has healed, even if the pain persists, pain behavior that was originally appropriate may become inappropriate and possibly even harmful. Although rest may be helpful after an acute injury, it may be counterproductive in chronic pain. People may lie around, become couch potatoes, gain weight, and get weaker. They begin to fear doing anything that might cause pain. They stay home, do not work, and get depressed. Their immobility causes their muscles to get weak and stiff, which contributes to greater impairment.

Psychological Diagnoses and Pain

The most common psychological problems in people with chronic pain are:

- Depression
- Anxiety disorder
- Substance abuse disorder
- Pain syndrome associated with both psychological factors and a general medical condition

Mental health professionals use specific criteria to make these medical diagnoses. However, there are other psychological problems that occur in people with chronic pain that are less specific, the most common of which are discussed later in this chapter and in chapter 16.

Depression

Many people with chronic pain get depressed, at least partly due to the losses resulting from their pain and impairment. Loss of income, loss of (or big changes in) relationships, and loss of job satisfaction may decrease a person's sense of self-worth and ability to enjoy life. Sadness, grief, and finally full-blown depression may follow. Eventually, the depression may take on a life of its own, even though it was triggered by pain. Depression is an illness that requires specific treatment—medications, psychotherapy, or both. People cannot just "snap out of it" any more than they can snap out of pneumonia.

There are two types of symptoms in depression—emotional and physical. The emotional symptoms involve feelings of sadness, helplessness, and hopelessness. Life's pleasures are lost. Negative thoughts and feelings—called ruminating thoughts—keep surfacing. The physical symptoms of depression vary. People with depression may experience sleep disturbances. They may have difficulty falling asleep, or they may wake early in the morning and be unable to fall back to sleep. Some people sleep excessively. They may lose their appetites and lose weight, although some people with depression overeat and gain weight. They may also lose the desire for sex, have low energy, and lose the ability to derive any pleasure from life.

Many times the diagnosis of depression is overlooked in patients with pain for several reasons. The symptoms of depression, such as those described above, may be attributed to the pain or to pain medications. Patients may not admit to the symptoms of depression because in our society there is a stigma attached to having a psychological problem. But the biggest reason may be that the diagnosis is just not considered by a doctor who is searching for physical causes of the problem. A good rule of thumb for doctors is that if the diagnosis of depression is even suspected, refer the patient to a psychologist or psychiatrist for consultation.

The relationship between pain and depression is complex. Again, the chicken and egg conundrum arises: Did the pain cause the depression or did the depression cause the pain? Depression that is caused by pain is called secondary depression or reactive depression. Depression that is independent of pain is called primary depression.

There is no doubt that depression, whether primary or secondary, can make pain worse. When pain and depression are both present, each must be treated if the patient is going to get better. The mind and body are too intimately related to hope that treating only the physical symptoms will lead to relief of the emotional problems. It bears repeating that depression must be treated, because once firmly established, it will not just get better if the pain improves and will also make the pain worse.

Anxiety Disorder

Anxiety is a state of worry, fearfulness, or uneasiness, often associated with fears and concerns about the future. It is not just the worry that is the problem; it is often the other symptoms that are so distressing. People with anxiety may have any or all of the following symptoms:

- An inner feeling of distress; feeling keyed-up or restless
- A general feeling of dis-ease; a sense that something is wrong, although it may not be clear exactly what is wrong

- Difficulty concentrating, racing thoughts, easily fatigued, or irritability. Problems falling asleep, staying asleep, or getting sleep that feels restorative
- Sensitivity to noises or crowds

Anxiety is not the same as the typical nervousness associated with an upcoming event, contest, or competition. Anxiety causes distress. Nervousness leads to action, and ends when the contest begins.

There are also physical symptoms associated with anxiety. For example, anxiety can lead to muscle tension. Since the neck is a vulnerable area, the muscles of the neck and jaw may tighten, which makes the neck pain even worse. Other physical symptoms of anxiety are:

- A sense of shortness of breath, often associated with the inability to take a full, complete, or satisfying deep breath
- Diarrhea, constipation, nausea, or vomiting
- Severe fatigue and the need to sleep all the time
- A feeling of a lump in the throat
- Tingling in both hands and feet
- A sense of skipped heartbeats or beats that feel stronger than usual

The anxiety that comes from neck pain usually is based on the fear of additional pain and the fear of reinjury. There are also worries about the future. One common element of these anxiety-producing emotions is the sense of powerlessness over the pain. There is probably no sensation as powerful as severe pain, and most people will do almost anything to avoid it. This fear of pain and the sense of loss of control over the pain leads to a marked limitation of activities of daily living in an effort to avoid more pain. People who experience pain for months or years may fear that it will never go away, that they will not be able to work, interact with friends or family, or ever have a normal life again. As with depression, anxiety originally due to pain can become a problem of its own, leading to sleep problems, negative thinking, and lowered tolerance to stress.

The good news is that anxiety can be treated. Stress reduction techniques, some of which are discussed in the next chapter, can help reduce anxiety and pain. Learning about the causes and treatment of the neck pain also helps by making it less of a mystery. Taking action to get better by exercising and working on body mechanics can do a great deal to overcome the feeling of powerlessness and loss of control. Taking charge and doing something active to get better, rather than remaining a victim of the pain, helps give back some sense of control and reduces the anxiety.

There are also medications that can help reduce anxiety. They are very effective in the short run, especially in the beginning stages of treatment. However, over the long-term, psychotherapy is probably better, because it can provide long-term solutions and coping mechanisms rather than just symptom relief.

Substance Abuse Disorder

Many people with pain take medications to try to seek some relief (see chapter 10). When used correctly, medications can be very helpful. Most medications used to treat pain, such as the opioid analgesics and sedatives, exert their effects in the brain. In vulnerable individuals, these medications can be harmful. Substance abuse disorder is a diagnostic term used to describe the psychological and physical problems produced by misuse of a medication, street drugs, or alcohol. There are many forms of substance abuse disorder, but dependence, addiction (including alcohol), and abuse are the ones seen most often in patients with pain.

Addiction is a disease defined as the "continued use of a psychoactive substance despite harm." The harm can be physical (cirrhosis due to alcohol), psychological (depression), or social (divorce or loss of a job). Addiction is always associated with loss of control over the drug or alcohol. When a person who is predisposed to an addictive disease is exposed to a potentially addictive substance, the addiction may become active. Another person who does not have addictive disease can take the same drug and suffer no harm. Addiction is quite uncommon in the treatment of pain, unless there was a preexisting addiction problem.

Many times, addiction is confused with dependence. Dependence is a physiological phenomenon that will occur in almost everyone who uses certain medications, alcohol, or street drugs long enough. Dependence means that if the substance were stopped abruptly, symptoms of withdrawal would occur. The type and intensity of withdrawal vary according to the substance used, the duration of use, and the dose.

Substance abuse is diagnosed when there are recurrent failures by the patient to fulfill major obligations in work, school, or homemaking that can be attributed to the use of a drug or alcohol. Other criteria include the sale of prescription pain medications, stealing medications from others, or stealing prescriptions from a doctor's office.

Most people who have been taking opioid pain relievers for many weeks or months become dependent. Dependence can make pain worse by leading to the phenomenon of "miniwithdrawal." In between doses of medication, the level of the pain reliever in the bloodstream falls, and if the level drops low enough, the patient has a "miniwithdrawal." The symptoms are not those of a full-blown withdrawal, with belly pain, diarrhea, and goose bumps. Instead, the major symptom is an increase in the pain, but there may be a craving for medications or a feeling of anxiety. These symptoms are sometimes referred to by pain specialists as "pseudo-addiction." Miniwithdrawal is seen commonly in patients who are somewhat dependent, and try to minimize the amount of medication they take. If they are taking their medication every six hours, but the medication only stays in the bloodstream four hours, they may suffer a miniwithdrawal for the last two hours, which results in a significant increase in the pain.

Addiction may make pain worse by unconsciously justifying the continued use of the drug. Because most people who are addicted are also dependent, a miniwithdrawal may also occur and make pain worse. The cycle of events often follows a predictable course. A person with addictive disease (or a predisposition for it) suffers a legitimate painful injury. A doctor prescribes a narcotic pain medication, which temporarily helps the pain, but also sets off a series of biochemical events in the brain that produces a pleasant feeling (euphoria). The euphoria becomes unconsciously connected to the medication and to justify taking the medication, the brain creates or worsens the pain. The patient then takes even more medication, which perpetuates and worsens the problem.

SECONDARY GAIN

Secondary gain is an unconscious psychological process that refers to any advantages a person gains as a consequence of his or her symptoms. In other words, a person achieves some benefit from neck pain that he or she could not get otherwise. There are some benefits to feeling bad.

There is no doubt that secondary gain exists, but it is dangerous to apply the secondary gain concept too broadly. If a person with neck pain does not get better quickly, and there is a lawsuit, it is too easy to attribute the poor outcome to the anticipated monetary gain from the lawsuit. Many doctors and lawyers assume that if there is money to be gained from being in pain, the injured person will continue to have pain. This does not mean the patient is faking. Secondary gain is unconscious, not deliberate fraud. It is true that some people who faked their injuries have obtained settlements, but these rare exceptions should not distort the picture for those with legitimate injuries.

When considering such an emotional topic, it is sometimes difficult to be logical, but looking at the scientific research on the subject can help. In 1961, H. Miller published an article, "Accident Neurosis," in the *British Medical Journal*, that supported the concept that patients could be "cured by verdict." Even though it was published forty years ago, this article continues to be used by defense lawyers and doctors to support the view that most people with prolonged neck pain after an injury either have a psychological cause for the pain (secondary gain) or are faking or exaggerating their pain and impairment to increase the chances of a large financial settlement. However, almost every study published since this oft-quoted article has reached the opposite conclusion by finding that most patients do not improve as a direct result of their cases being settled.

There are three types of direct financial rewards for an injury—workers' compensation benefits, private disability payments, and personal injury litigation. When a person is injured on the job, workers' compensation insurance pays the costs of medical care, and the injured worker also collects workers' compensation disability insurance. There is no doubt that injured workers do not do as well as others with the same type of injuries. Injured workers take longer to recover and have lower return-to-work rates than people who were not injured on the job.

There is no scientific information regarding the effects of long-term disability payments from private disability insurance. However, there is a large body of scientific information about the effects of personal injury litigation. Almost every scientist who has studied the effects of personal injury litigation on recovery from injury has concluded that lawsuits themselves do not prevent recovery. This may seem contrary to common sense, but that is what the evidence shows. People who are injured in car accidents and who develop whiplash are often criticized as being fakers or just out for the money. Almost everyone I have treated would gladly trade every bit of settlement money for pain relief and a return to a normal life.

Malingering

Malingering means faking or pretending to have an injury, pain, or incapacity. Malingering is a way to avoid work or other duties, get disability payments, or win a legal settlement after a real or alleged injury. It is not a psychological problem—it is fraud. In every society, there are people who try to take advantage of any situation, including the medical and legal systems, for their own personal gain. There are reports of fraud rings of people who stage auto accidents, slips, or falls. They may even be in league with lawyers who team with fraudulent doctors or chiropractors who generate fraudulent injury reports. These cases make the headlines, but they constitute a very small minority of all injury lawsuits. Yet, these few bad apples have left a very negative impression on the public, lawyers, and doctors.

It is not possible to know for certain if a person has pain, because pain is invisible. Therefore, doctors, lawyers, judges, and juries must determine if a patient who reports pain is truthful. Some people with fake injuries can be quite convincing, while others with real and painful injuries may seem disingenuous. There are no definitive tests for pain that can tell if a patient is not truthful. However, usually there will be inconsistencies in the history, examination, diagnostic tests, and responses to treatment that will suggest something is amiss. Experienced physicians usually will be able to determine when a patient is malingering.

CHILDHOOD ABUSE AND CHRONIC PAIN

Each of us has a unique character structure and personality that has been formed over many years. We are born with our own unique genetic predisposition for our personalities, which are then shaped by the events of our lives. The genetic makeup is like the painter's blank canvas. There are many types, sizes, and textures of canvases, and there are probably an infinite number of genetic predispositions for personalities. The painter creates a work of art by applying layers of paint to the canvas, just as each event of our lives inscribes itself upon our psychological makeup. Over time, the canvas changes as new layers of paint are applied. The final quality of the work depends on the type of canvas and the paints applied, just as our psychological character is based on our genetic makeup and the psychological effects of people and events that have shaped our lives. As a result, some of us are psychologically strong and able to weather adverse events, but others are more psychologically vulnerable to stresses such as pain.

During the years that our psychological character is being formed, it is vulnerable to severe psychological trauma. Childhood abuse is a particularly powerful trauma that can severely disrupt the formation of a healthy character structure. Most of the research on the relationship between pain and childhood

abuse has dealt with physical and sexual abuse. It is well established that adults who have been abused as children have a
much higher prevalence of headaches, low back pain, and in
women, pelvic pain. We have already seen that pain is both a
sensory and emotional experience and that the mind and body
are intimately connected. It appears that people who have had
an abusive childhood are at high risk for chronic pain. Their
normal template has been damaged. Such people have been
called "pain prone" by the physician Dr. George Engel. Their
pain is real. It is just that psychological factors play a much big-
ger role than usual.

In research at our clinic, we have investigated the relationship between childhood abuses and low back pain. We have
shown that at least five risk factors—physical abuse, sexual
abuse, abandonment (not simple divorce), psychological abuse,
and addictive disease in one or both caregivers—put a person at
greater risk of developing chronic pain following injury. The
more types of childhood traumas a person has experienced, the
more disrupted the template and the more difficult it is for the
patient to recover from pain. While we have not conducted
formal research in people with neck pain, our impression is
that the same factors hold true. An abusive childhood does not
cause pain, but it makes it much more difficult to recover.

When I see patients who are not recovering from a neck
injury fairly quickly, I often obtain a psychological consultation. I am not surprised to hear there is a history of abuse,
and psychological factors are contributing to the pain and
delayed recovery. In fact, in our research, one-third of our
patients who had been abused had never disclosed it before to
anyone!

It is important to place the role of childhood abuse in
perspective. Many people have adapted to the severely dysfunc-

tional childhood events and gone on to be happy and productive. However, others have become dysfunctional. Obviously, we cannot change the past, but we can work on the effects of the abuse through psychotherapy, and possibly relieve some of the pain and distress of the physical injury as well.

17

Psychological Problems and Chronic Pain: What You Can Do

Psychological factors play a role in almost every case of chronic pain, although the type and intensity of psychological factors differ from person to person. In the previous chapter, I reviewed the medical aspects of the psychology of chronic pain. In this chapter, I present the more personal components of psychological problems and provide action steps that each person can take to feel better.

It is worthwhile to review the definition of pain proposed by the International Association for the Study of Pain. Pain is "an unpleasant *sensory* and *emotional* experience associated with actual or potential tissue damage or described in terms of tissue damage" (italics mine). By definition, then, pain always has some form and degree of emotional content. In some people, the emotional contribution to the pain may be minimal, but in others it may predominate.

Failing to recognize, accept, understand, and treat the psychological components of chronic pain is one of the greatest roadblocks to recovery. Both patients and doctors need to accept that although psychological factors may at times be difficult to face, the goal is to get better, no matter what it takes.

Many people with chronic pain believe that if (or when) the pain gets better, all of life's other problems will disappear, but this is rarely the case. However, even if psychological issues developed as a result of the pain, they may become independent of the pain. If the psychological problems are not treated in parallel with the underlying physical problem, the person with chronic pain will not get well. When chronic pain takes hold, the pain becomes a black hole, and all of life's problems seem to be pulled into it. Many people with chronic pain tend to blame everything on the pain—problems with relationships, finances, insurance companies, employers, and doctors. But life is filled with challenges for everyone, whether they have pain or not. When a person feels a loss of control over pain, they may also feel a loss of control over many of life's ordinary issues.

The first step toward getting better is to recognize any psychological problems that are present, admit they are there, and seek treatment. The cycle of helplessness and hopelessness makes the future look bleak. The techniques described in this chapter, coupled with medications and psychotherapy when necessary, may be helpful in breaking the downhill spiral.

PSYCHOLOGICAL COMPONENTS OF CHRONIC PAIN

In chapter 16, I discussed the major psychological diagnoses—depression, anxiety, and substance abuse—from the medical perspective. This chapter addresses these and other parts of the pain experience from a more personal perspective.

Depression

Depression occurs in as many as 45 percent of people with chronic low back pain, and it is probably almost as common in neck pain. Depression can make pain worse, and also causes symptoms of its own—sleep disturbances, weight change, loss of energy and libido—which are described in chapter 16. Symptoms of depression may begin as soon as three months after the start of a pain problem, but they usually take longer to appear. Obviously, not all people with chronic pain get depressed. It may be that some people are predisposed to depression by virtue of their genetics, underlying psychological makeup, prior psychological problems, or prior experiences with loss and grief.

People with neck pain who get depressed harbor feelings of helplessness and hopelessness. Helplessness develops in part because nothing has worked to lessen the pain. The person in pain feels as if he or she has lost control, not only over the pain, but over many of the normal activities of daily living. He or she feels at the mercy of the pain, helpless to do anything about it. Once this "learned helplessness" has been established, treatment with individual or group psychotherapy and medications for the depression must be included with rehabilitation for the neck pain.

Hopelessness often follows helplessness. A patient who sees doctor after doctor, but continues to have pain, may feel there is no hope, which makes depression even worse. Eventually, in addition to the sadness and other mood changes, the physical symptoms appear as well.

Depression deserves treatment, preferably by a mental health professional who can assess the condition and plan the best treatment. However, several self-help techniques that are described later in this chapter have been proven effective for some people.

Anxiety

Anxiety is a fear often associated with an inner nervous feeling in the gut that is usually about the future. It occurs in as many as 17 percent of patients with chronic low back pain, and may be almost as common in neck pain. Anxiety can be caused by worry about something specific, or it can be more generalized. The symptoms of anxiety include irritability, sleeplessness, short temper, and fear. They are discussed in more detail in chapter 16. When severe, anxiety can interfere with the ability to function normally.

Although anxiety is an emotional disorder, it may be expressed physically, even if there are no psychological symptoms. The physical symptoms of anxiety are discussed in chapter 16, and include rapid heart rate, sweating, abdominal pain, or diarrhea. Some patients have an increase in muscle tension that makes pain even worse. Then, in turn, the increased pain can worsen the anxiety, and a vicious cycle is established.

Anxiety should not be ignored for several reasons: it can make pain worse; it can cause a deterioration in function; and it may not go away without treatment regardless of what happens to the pain. We now have effective treatments for anxiety including the relaxation techniques described in the following sections, psychotherapy, and medications.

Medication and Alcohol Abuse

The overuse or abuse of prescription medications, such as opioid analgesics and antianxiety drugs, may become a problem in patients with chronic pain. These drugs can be very helpful when used properly, but overuse or abuse may be dangerous and can even make pain worse. Although they may not realize it, some people use alcohol, pain medications, or sedatives to medicate or suppress their unpleasant emotions. They may think they are taking medications to relieve their pain, but they are actually using these substances to "self-medicate" their unpleasant feelings. Unfortunately, although the alcohol or medications may make a person feel better initially, soon the substances make the feelings and moods even worse.

Alcohol abuse may be more prevalent in people with chronic pain than in the general population, but there are no exact figures available. There is a complex relationship between alcohol and chronic pain. Some people who drink, especially those who drink excessively, may be more prone to accidents and injuries. An intoxicated person may feel less inhibited, take foolish chances, and may be more likely to get hurt. Being "high" might even temporarily raise pain threshold and tolerance, which may lead to poor injury recognition, and increase the risk of further damage. Drinkers are more likely than nondrinkers to be involved in car, bicycle, and boating accidents.

Some people drink alcohol to relieve pain, because alcohol does have some analgesic qualities. Alcohol can temporarily calm anxiety, it is freely available, and for the most part, it is culturally acceptable.

Alcohol overuse and abuse pose many dangers for the person with chronic neck pain. Working around potentially dangerous equipment when drinking may be especially risky because a new accident may reinjure an already vulnerable neck. Chronic alcohol use can cause depression. Alcohol can increase the potency of some prescription and over-the-counter medications, especially opioid analgesics and sedatives, which can increase the risk of dangerous side effects. For example, acetaminophen, the ingredient in Tylenol, is much more likely to cause liver damage in people who drink heavily.

At least 10 percent of the general population are alcoholic, and so at least 10 percent of people with neck pain will also be alcoholic. One definition of alcohol addiction is continued and compulsive use despite harm. The harm can be physical (liver damage, reinjury of the neck), social (loss of job, divorce), or emotional (depression). Patients with chronic pain should be very careful to avoid using excess alcohol to deal with the pain. Some patients may require treatment for alcoholism.

Pain Behaviors

Pain usually leads to some actions or reactions, which are called pain behaviors. Pain behaviors can be purposeful or unconscious, appropriate and beneficial, or inappropriate and harmful, depending on the circumstances. Pain behaviors that are appropriate for acute pain to foster healing may become detrimental for chronic pain and lead to deconditioning and depression.

Some pain behaviors are learned unconsciously by a process called reinforcement. Most of us are familiar with the famous experiments of Pavlov in which he taught dogs to salivate at the sound of a bell. He began by ringing a bell and then feeding the dogs, who would salivate naturally at the sight of food. Over time, the dogs would associate the sound of the bell with feeding, and would begin to salivate just at the sound of the bell. The dogs had learned to associate a behavior (salivating) with the sound of a bell. Similar mechanisms operate in people—certain behaviors can become linked to increased pain, and then the behaviors occur even without the pain, particularly in any set or setting that might have provoked the pain in the past.

In humans, rewards (something positive that occurs as a result of the pain) may serve to reinforce pain behaviors. Some people do not ordinarily get needed attention from spouses, children, friends, or coworkers. Then, after they are injured, they suddenly get that attention, and if there were no pain, there would be no special attention. Such attention may be helpful for dealing with the acute pain of a recent injury, but may serve to reinforce learned behaviors leading to chronic pain and further inactivity. Family members may offer a massage, cook or serve dinner, or bring medications to the person with chronic pain—all forms of attention not otherwise available. But soon the extra attention—the reward for being in pain—has to be justified unconsciously and so the pain must continue.

Some rewards take the form of avoiding something unpleasant, such as a bad job or a bad supervisor. Because of pain, the injured worker may stay home, and not have to deal with a bad job situation. Soon, the worker's unconscious mind has linked staying at home (and thereby avoiding the unpleasantness) to being in pain, and to justify staying home from work, there must be pain. Even if the injury has healed, the pain must continue or the worker would have to return to work. The pain is conditioned into the mind. It has been shown that injured workers with legitimate injuries, but who dislike their jobs or supervisors, recover more slowly from their injuries than employees who like their jobs and supervisors. The pain of the injury is an unconscious way to avoid an unpleasant job situation. This should not, however, be confused with faking. Learned pain is a psychological and unconscious process.

Other people may also reinforce conditioned behaviors. Doctors can inadvertently reinforce the learned abnormal pain behavior by giving an injured worker a disability excuse for time off work when it is not totally necessary. They may prescribe medications that eventually do more harm than good.

They may recommend bed rest rather than exercise. Employers may also reinforce abnormal pain behavior. Rather than provide modified duty, they may not take workers back unless they are "100 percent."

Insurers may also reinforce abnormal pain behavior. They may make surveillance videotapes of an injured worker or accident victim. After an insurer has done this to some workers, word spreads. Then an injured worker is afraid of doing even minimal work around the home for fear of being taped and losing disability or insurance benefits.

Sleep Disturbances

Many people with chronic neck pain have some form of sleep problems. They may have difficulties falling asleep, staying asleep, or getting sleep that is restful and restorative. It is very important to get a good night's sleep, since poor sleep can contribute to increased pain, decreased function, and less ability to cope with pain.

Most people blame poor sleep on the pain, but there are other reasons for poor sleep as well. Sleep disturbance is one of the symptoms of depression, particularly early morning awakening with difficulty falling back to sleep, and sleep that is nonrestorative. Anxiety disorders can also disturb sleep, especially if there are recurring intrusive thoughts about pain, finances, family matters, and the future. Other factors that influence sleep include diet, exercise, and activity level.

Sleep specialists have developed strategies to help deal with insomnia. Perhaps because these recommendations seem so obvious, people with sleep difficulties often ignore them. However, some of these simple things can make big differences and are:

- Avoid napping during the daytime, even when tired.
- Go to bed at the same time each night, and get out of bed the same time every morning, even if the night's sleep was not good.
- Exercise regularly, but avoid exercising within two hours of going to bed.
- Use the bed only for sleep or sex, not for reading or watching television (unless reading in bed or watching television puts you to sleep).
- Experiment with different bedroom temperatures to find the range that is best.
- Avoid going to bed with a full stomach—allow at least three hours between the last meal and going to bed.
- Consider investing in a special well-designed mattress and special neck pillow (see chapter 9 and appendix B). Water-filled pillows or foam pillows appear to provide the best sleep, and adjustable air mattresses can also provide some benefit.
- Use relaxation techniques to help you fall asleep.

If relaxation and the other self-help techniques discussed in the following sections are not effective, prescription medications can be very valuable. The best drugs appear to be the sedating antidepressants such as amitriptyline, nortriptyline, doxepin, or trazodone. Pure sleep medications are not as useful because they do not help pain. However, zolpidem (Ambien), a newer sleep medication, is effective, has fewer side effects than the older drugs, and rarely causes early morning hangover. Melatonin, a human hormone that plays a role in regulating our internal clocks, has been found to help some people sleep. It can be bought over the counter, and has few side effects.

Negative Thoughts

It is virtually impossible to ignore pain. Everyone with chronic pain thinks about it throughout the day. Unfortunately, these negative thoughts often take a downward spiral and can themselves become a problem. At first, people tend to analyze the frequency, duration, intensity, and, perhaps most important, the meaning of their pain. They might analyze what causes it and what makes it better. Eventually, the excess analysis turns to paralysis. The thoughts become less analytical and more critical. The negative thoughts may become intrusive. Beliefs set in that the pain will never end, that life will never be the same, and that there is no hope.

After a while, the thinking changes again, and becomes even less controlled. A person may become hypervigilant—constantly scanning the body to look or feel for any pains, even those that have nothing to do with the original neck pain. This extra attention to the pain and worrying about it makes it worse. The thoughts become progressively more negative, and eventually the pain becomes a black hole into which all of life's problems are sucked.

These negative thoughts must be changed. It is very useful to begin by taking note of each negative thought, and writing it down, as described in the section later in this chapter on journal writing. Then it is useful to examine each negative thought to look for ways to change the pattern of negative thinking and the patterns, thoughts, and ideas that bring them on. *The Chronic Pain Control Workbook*, by Ellen Catalano and Kim Hardin, offers valuable suggestions for looking at negative thoughts and changing them (see appendix A, "Selected Readings").

Fears

Some of the things people with chronic neck pain fear are that the pain will never go away, the pain will get worse, and that their necks are so fragile they will be reinjured easily. The last two may result in the avoidance of activities that might aggravate the pain or cause reinjury. When these fears are out of proportion to the reality of the risks, they may lead to significant and unnecessary decreases in function.

There is a big difference between unrealistic fears and reasonable concerns. It is very appropriate to be concerned about neck pain, and to avoid those things that make it worse. It is also appropriate to eliminate or modify unnecessary activities to minimize the chances of a flare. However, life goes on. It is important to evaluate fears and concerns and to develop a reasonable activity plan. We can use rational thinking to overcome irrational thoughts.

Family Issues

Family issues are also complex, and may involve both the family of origin and the current family. The ways in which parents dealt with their own illnesses, injuries, and emotions strongly influence the ways their adult children deal with similar problems. In addition, as described previously, the ways spouses, children, and parents react and relate to the person with chronic neck pain may accentuate the pain and pain behavior of the injured person.

Families may grow apart when one member has chronic pain. The injured person may begin to focus more attention inward and lose interest in the family. The family, in turn, loses interest in the person with pain. The healthy spouse grows tired of all the extra work, and may feel unappreciated and overwhelmed. Couples may fight, and eventually grow apart. Family therapy is often necessary to break these patterns, and may work best if it is begun at an early phase of the illness.

Cultural Issues

Cultural influences may also come into play with chronic pain. There are good research data to show that people of different cultures react differently to the same types of pain. Although these are generalities, people of European ancestry tend to experience significantly less pain after a tooth is pulled than do persons of Afro-American or Latino descent. In this same study, Asians tended to experience slightly more pain than those of European descent.

The explanation for the differences is not clear, but may be either genetic or acquired culturally. It does not change the treatment of painful disorders, but it is useful to bear in mind. All other things being equal, based on ethnic or cultural variables, some people may be predisposed to have more pain, and therefore more impairment, than others.

"Tension Myositis Syndrome"

Neck pain, low back pain, and headache are three of the most common problems that bring patients to doctors. Some people become frustrated with the health care system because they do not get better, and become attracted to treatments popularized in the media (see chapter 14). They may turn toward the simple answers offered by self-declared experts who promote their miracle cures and their theories to support them.

Dr. John Sarno at NYU is a physician who has written several books on back pain and other muscle, joint, and soft tissue pains. He believes that virtually all patients with back or neck pain are suffering from "tension myositis syndrome," or TMS, a term that he coined and has popularized in his books and media appearances. His theory is that back and neck pain are almost always due to a change in the state of muscles and nerves. He states that emotional tension causes a reaction in the nervous system that causes constriction of blood vessels to certain muscles and nerves, which are then deprived of proper blood flow. The muscles develop spasm and hurt. Dr. Sarno says that objective findings (such as disc herniations, displaced vertebrae, or other structural disorders) are not important, and have nothing to do with the pain.

Dr. Sarno goes on to say that the acceptance of TMS as the cause for the pain by the person with the pain will, in and of itself, result in a reduction or elimination of pain. He believes there is no need for exercise, and moreover that any value from exercise is a placebo effect. He sees no role for relaxation training, yoga, or biofeedback. He feels psychotherapy can be useful, but is not essential, because it is the mere acceptance that there is an underlying emotional issue that makes the pain fade, not the treatment of the emotional issue. Dr. Sarno claims to have cured more than 85 percent of his patients, and those who did not get better failed because they did not accept his theory for the cause of their pain.

Unfortunately, the studies Dr. Sarno has performed to justify his conclusions do not meet rigorous scientific standards for proof, and have never been presented to a group of scientists for review. Instead, they are his personal opinion. In addition, it is naïve to think there is a single cause for every patient with back or neck pain. No other doctor or researcher has been able to get the same amazing results with any other form of treatment. For all these reasons, at this time it is not reasonable to accept this popular theory. However, as described in the sections above and in chapter 16, psychological or emotional problems are very important in the genesis and continuation of chronic neck pain in some people.

PSYCHOLOGICAL SELF-TREATMENTS FOR CHRONIC PAIN

Many people with chronic pain read about the psychological aspects of pain, and think that, although the subject is interesting, it has little to do with them. Most people are much more interested in the physical aspects of the pain and the physical treatments. They may glance at the suggestions for psychological treatments, but decide not to try them. However, all chronic pain has both physical and psychological components, although the percentage of each varies from one person to the next. In a person with a mild, annoying pain, there is little need to consider the role of possible psychological components, but in a person with severe pain and impairment, if psychological factors are not addressed, treatment is not going to work. Virtually all experts in pain management agree that psychological factors are often very important and must be considered seriously.

No single treatment is appropriate for every person. I would suggest each person try a few things to see what feels best. A combination of relaxation training and journal writing would be a minimum program.

Knowledge as Power

Much of the anxiety, helplessness, and hopelessness that surrounds chronic neck pain is fueled by fears of the unknown. One of the purposes of this book is to provide the knowledge to demystify neck pain and allay those fears. Some people visit doctor after doctor, but no diagnosis is ever made and no treatments work. This apparent failure of modern medicine to successfully diagnose and treat makes the problem seem a mystery, which compounds the fear. If expert doctors are not able to figure out what is wrong, the future appears bleak.

This can change. The specialties of spine medicine and surgery are relatively new, but research in this area has advanced our understanding of neck pain tremendously in the past decade. Much of the current information was not even known when some doctors who still practice were in medical school. It is up to the person with pain to learn as much as possible, and to find a doctor who is up-to-date with current thinking, research, and treatment of painful spinal disorders. Knowledge is power—power over pain.

Overcoming Unreasonable Fears

Many times, doctors do not consider their patients' fears seriously. The doctor understands the condition, and knows whether it is serious. The doctor may assume the patient also knows the neck problem is not likely to get worse, nor lead to nerve damage or paralysis. So what's the fuss? But doctors may forget that patients do not have the same knowledge and experience. They only know their pain, and often fear the worst. To compound the matter, the doctor recommends exercise and a return to normal activities, but the patient silently questions this advice. How can I act normally if there is so much pain? Won't I get worse? They conclude that the doctor is wrong, decide not to follow the advice, and move on to another doctor or alternative health care practitioner.

These seemingly disparate views of how to get better can be reconciled, because both are true. Doctors are correct to emphasize exercise, body mechanics, and normalization of activities, because in the long-term, this helps people get better. However, it is also true that activities done improperly cause more pain. So it is imperative that doctors teach their patients how to be active, and explain things carefully before sending them off with reassurances. They must refer the patients to physical therapists or trainers who will supervise the return to activities. These explanations will go a long way to overcoming unreasonable fears. In addition, psychotherapy, pain groups, and information all contribute to overcoming many of the fears.

However, patients have a responsibility as well. When they have questions or doubts about their doctors' recommendations, they should ask specific questions and ask for recommendations for books or Web sites that provide additional information. It is helpful when patients bring a short list—a long list is overwhelming to a doctor—of questions to the appointment.

We have learned throughout our lives that pain means something is wrong, and if there is pain, it is important to rest the injured part until the pain decreases. We have also learned, perhaps unconsciously, that if pain continues, it must be because the injury has not healed. We learned that "hurt equals harm," but this conventional wisdom applies to acute pain, not chronic pain. In most instances, the best thing to do for chronic pain is to remain active. It may be difficult to accept this when it hurts, because on the surface, it makes little sense. But it is true. Chronic pain is so different from acute pain that the lessons we have learned no longer apply.

People in chronic pain must use their own critical thinking to override their intuition and old learning in this case. They must use their willpower to get better. As people progress with their exercises and body mechanics, they will be able to do more and more without making their pain worse. Eventually, the nervous system gets reprogrammed and the pain decreases.

How to Return to Normal Activities

When pain leads to inactivity, muscles weaken and motivation to get active again decreases. In order to get better, the muscles must be reconditioned. In fact, they must get stronger than they were before the pain began. An injured football player who has surgery does not return to the field immediately. He begins an aggressive rehabilitation program to strengthen muscles that have grown weak from inactivity. The athlete returns to play only when the muscles are strong.

The same is true for a person with neck pain. The return to normal activities must occur in a graduated manner. It should start slowly and increase slowly as well. The increases in activity must be done according to a predetermined plan, not according to the level of pain.

To begin to return to normal activities, it is best to select an activity, such as sitting at the computer, that you can do for at least a short period of time. Then choose an amount of time from your recent experience that you can spend at this task without precipitating a flare. It is important to be truthful with yourself. It does not matter where you start, it matters where you end. One method is to sit at the computer for the chosen amount of time. Set a timer—do not estimate. Once you reach your goal, you can stop, get up, and move around. You are done.

Then, during the same day and the next morning, see how you feel. It is common to feel slightly worse, but not to feel much worse. If your pain is not worse the next day, increase your activity by 10 percent. If you are slightly worse, increase by only 5 percent. If you are much worse, decrease by 10 percent, but do not give up. Follow this pattern each day, increasing or decreasing by 5 percent or 10 percent, depending on your response to the prior day's activities.

As an example, if you worked at a task for ten minutes on day one, and were no worse the next day, then on day two you would increase your time to eleven minutes. (Here's how to do the math: Ten minutes is equal to 600 seconds. Ten percent of that is 60 seconds, so 60 seconds is added to the original 600 seconds, for a total of 660 seconds, or eleven minutes.) On the third day, your time spent sitting at the computer will be 726 seconds (the day two quota of 660 seconds, plus 10 percent of 660, which would be 660 plus 66 = 726). Obviously, you can round off these numbers. The increases are very small at first, but they get larger after about a week, just like the miracle of compound interest.

RELAXATION TECHNIQUES

Relaxation techniques can help relieve anxiety, and the physical part of the stresses of daily life. Relaxation can help painful and overworked muscles relax, and may provide some degree of pain relief. Strange as it may seem, learning to relax takes work and practice. However, once mastered, relaxation techniques are very useful for the treatment of chronic neck pain. Not all techniques work for everyone. I will discuss several techniques that are practical, easy to learn, and potentially helpful. After trying several, use those that are most helpful to you.

Deep Breathing

Deep breathing has been used for thousands of years to combat stress, ease tension, and produce feelings of calm and relaxation. Deep breathing is an important part of almost every meditation and stress reduction program. For most people with chronic neck pain, deep breathing can be a valuable part of treatment, both as part of a program to keep pain and stress under control, and to treat acute flares while using the neck rest position for neck first aid (see chapter 7).

Deep breathing is easy to learn and can be done anywhere and in almost any position. It is probably best to learn the technique lying down, because it is easiest on the neck. Assume the neck rest position (see chapter 7) by lying on your back on a firm surface such as a carpeted floor. Bend your hips and knees to about 45 degrees, but keep both feet flat on the floor. Place a tightly rolled hand towel under your neck near the base of your skull. Place your hands palm down on the floor along the sides. Make sure your shoulders are relaxed, and keep your eyes open but unfocused.

Take a slow, deep, full breath through your nose, then let air out slowly through your mouth, perhaps pursing your lips to control and slow the release of air. Focus on the muscles of your neck and shoulders and feel them begin to relax. With each breath, let the muscles relax still more. After one or two minutes, move one hand to a place halfway between your belly button and chest bone. Allow your breathing to gently push your hand up toward the ceiling. With each breath, your tension eases. Continue this exercise for ten to fifteen minutes, and do it at least twice a day.

Relaxation Training, Meditation, and Rhythmic Breathing

There are many words to describe relaxation training, including meditation, which has become quite popular lately. Meditation is not a religion, although it is a part of many religious practices. Many of the same exercises that have been used for centuries in meditation are similar to those used in relaxation training. There are many forms of meditation, but one of the best is "following your breath." Although this form of training is usually done seated, you can also do it lying down. However, when lying down and meditating, there is a tendency to fall asleep, and that is why sitting is usually preferred. It is important to use good sitting posture, perhaps with a chair that has head and neck support.

The technique begins by getting into a comfortable position. Begin by breathing normally through your nose. Gently lower your eyelids somewhat, keeping your eyes open but unfocused. Move your attention to the tip of your nose and begin to pay attention to your breath as it enters and exits your nose. Then, while you inhale, count slowly to ten. Then, as you exhale, count to ten again. If your mind starts to wander or you find yourself daydreaming, refocus and start again. You can do this meditation for ten to fifteen minutes each day. It is a powerful relaxation and stress reduction tool, which can also help ease the pain of tension for many people.

Progressive Muscle Relaxation

Progressive muscle relaxation (PMR) is an excellent technique to help with pain that comes from tense neck muscles. In many patients, the neck muscles remain in a state of tension because they are injured, too weak to hold the head in proper position, or kept in awkward positions for long durations. PMR can help the muscles relax and decrease some of the pain. PMR can be useful both for prevention and as part of neck first aid. It is also useful to perform PMR before doing the deep-breathing relaxation exercises. The basis for PMR is overtightening a group of muscles and then relaxing them.

The exercise begins by lying on the floor in the neck rest position. Focus your attention on your right hand. Gradually form a fist, progressively tightening it until you are squeezing very hard. As you hold your hand in a tight fist, notice that the tightness is moving up your arm. Hold the clenched fist for thirty seconds or until you feel your forearm begin to cramp or burn. Then relax your hand completely. Then do the same exercise with your other hand. Repeat each side three times.

The next PMR exercise is for the muscles at the base of your neck and upper back. This exercise can be done either lying down, sitting in a chair, or on a stool. Start in either a good sitting neutral spine position or in the neck rest position. Bring both shoulders up toward your jaw as far as you can. Hold the position for fifteen to thirty seconds or until you feel slight pain in your shoulder muscles, then relax, letting your shoulders fall to their natural position. Continue your deep breathing, and then repeat this exercise three times.

The PMR exercise for the muscles between the shoulder blades should leave you with a feeling that the tension has gone out of your neck muscles. Once again, this exercise can be done either lying on the floor in the neck rest position or seated. If you are doing it lying down, place a tightly rolled dish towel vertically between your shoulder blades. The neck rest towel can remain under your neck. If you are sitting, get in a good neutral posture. Then move your shoulder blades toward each other until you feel tension in the muscles. Hold the position until the tension becomes slightly painful, and then relax your muscles. Repeat this exercise three times.

The last PMR exercise is for the muscles in the back of the neck. It is done lying in the neck rest position, with no towel between your shoulder blades, but still using the neck rest towel behind your neck. Place a washcloth or sponge behind your head. Then simply push the back of your head against the washcloth or sponge for fifteen seconds or until the tension builds up. Then relax your muscles. Repeat the exercise three times. This PMR exercise is the same as one of the exercises that is used to strengthen the muscles of the back of your neck (see chapter 8).

Journal Writing

There are many reasons for a person with chronic neck pain to keep a journal. It is one way to discover which activities cause pain to worsen. It is a good way to get in touch with any unrecognized feelings about your pain, to see the impact the pain has on your life, and to begin to get these thoughts and feelings out. Expressing your feelings and thoughts may also help relieve some of the stress that builds up due to the pain, so journal writing can be psychologically therapeutic. I would encourage every person with chronic pain to keep a journal. Write at least once a day, and more often if it feels right.

For someone dealing with chronic pain, it may be useful to make different types of entries. You can keep separate sections in one journal or use different journals—one for feelings and thoughts, one to write about stressful events, and one for the diary of activities of daily living. Each type of journal writing serves a different purpose in the healing process.

Writing About Feelings and Thoughts

When you have chronic pain, it is important to get in touch with your feelings and emotions, think about them, and interpret what they might mean to you. This requires time to pause, take note of your feelings, and then reflect on them, a process which many people find difficult.

One of the roles of psychotherapy is to help you do these same things. However, many people do not have access to a psychotherapist, or are uncomfortable discussing intimate aspects of their lives with a stranger. One effective way to overcome these obstacles and still have a means to express feelings is to keep a journal—a diary of personal feelings and thoughts.

Every person with chronic pain has some form of emotional response. There may be denial, anger, blame, fear, anxiety, depression, and a great deal of suffering. Pent-up feelings can make the pain fester, like a boil. Getting the feelings out—on paper or to a therapist—can be therapeutic, and most people feel better when they do this. When you express your feelings on a regular basis, there can be significant improvement in pain.

There is no correct way to keep a journal. The most important things are to write regularly, honestly, and without self-criticism. The journal is for you, the journal writer, not for others to read. Write as if nobody else will ever see your journal. Write whatever comes up. Don't worry about spelling or grammar—they are not important for your journal. It is often good to start by writing for ten minutes at about the same time every day. If there is more to say, sit longer. Each entry is new, and does not need to have anything to do with prior entries. Expressing your inner thoughts and feelings is all that matters.

Writing About Daily Activities

In this type of journal writing, activities are recorded day by day and hour by hour. The goal is to discover which activities make your pain better or worse. It is best to make a detailed activity list in four columns. In column one, record the date and time. In column two, note your pain level before the activity on a scale of 0 (where 0 is no pain) to 10 (where pain is as bad as you could ever imagine). In column three, write down your pain level after finishing the activity. In column four, write down any ideas that come to you while you are doing the other columns. Be sure that periodically you review your journal to find any patterns or trends.

When writing about the activities that change your pain, it is important to record something every hour or so. If your pain level is particularly high (perhaps a 6 or greater), it may be useful to look at the activities of the prior hours or days for clues to the cause of the flare.

Writing About Stressful Events

By now, it should be obvious that there is at least some connection between your pain and emotions. Things that have occurred in your past as well as things that have occurred recently can affect your emotions and your pain. It can be very helpful in terms of pain relief to get these feelings out. This can be done with a psychotherapist, but another way to accomplish this privately, without the need for professional help, is to write about stressful events. Writing about stressful events for just twenty minutes, three times a week, for four to six weeks, has been proven to improve breathing in people with asthma and reduce inflammation and pain in people with rheumatoid arthritis. Although there has been no research about the effect of writing about stressful events in people with neck pain, it appears that there can be improvements in pain through the use of writing, and there is certainly no risk.

Writing about stressful events differs from writing about feelings and emotions because it is a little more structured. The technique is simple. Find a place in private to sit with pen and paper. There should be no interruptions, and the phone should be turned off. Set a timer for twenty minutes, during which you write about the most stressful experiences you have ever had. Again, do not be concerned about spelling, grammar, or neatness, because nobody else will read this work.

Repeat this process the next day, and then get in the habit of writing about stressful events at least three times a week. You can continue writing more about the same events or you can choose to write about different stresses. When it feels right and you are comfortable with the process of writing about yourself and your life, begin to write about pain, fears, and emotions. In many instances, you may experience a decrease in pain, stress, and anxiety.

MEDICATIONS

Medications have been discussed in detail in chapter 10. In this section, I will briefly review the medications used for the psychological problems of chronic pain.

Antidepressants

Antidepressants are useful for people with chronic pain to treat depression, sleep disturbance, pain that arises from nerve damage, and the neck pain itself. In general terms, there are two very broad classes of antidepressants: the cyclic antidepressants and the selective serotonin reuptake inhibitors (SSRIs). These medications can be very helpful when the proper drug is used. I have discussed the use of antidepressants for pain in chapter 10, but I will briefly review their use for the treatment of depression here. Remember that antidepressants are not a substitute for psychotherapy, or for needed changes in behavior, negative thoughts, or lifestyle. Instead, antidepressants should be considered as just one part of an overall treatment program.

In depression, there are biochemical changes in the brain. It does not matter if the depression is unrelated to pain or if it is caused by the pain and impairment. The two major biochemicals that are decreased in depression are serotonin and norepinephrine. The antidepressants work by restoring the biochemistry of the brain (and perhaps other nerves) to normal. They are not like amphetamines, or cocaine, which cause unnatural biochemical states.

It appears that a decreased level of serotonin is the major biochemical abnormality seen in depression, and the SSRIs are extremely effective in restoring the serotonin levels back toward normal. All of the SSRIs share this mechanism of action and all have similar side effects. The antidepressants fluoxetine (Prozac), sertraline (Zoloft), paroxetine (Paxil), citalopram (Celexa), and nefazodone (Serzone) are usually very effective in this regard. The choice of drug is based on the experiences of your doctor, your other medical problems, and your prior experiences with these medications. Some people will respond to one and not another, and will have side effects with one drug and not another. It may require several trials to find the most effective drug with the fewest side effects.

When these drugs work, most of the symptoms of depression, including depressed mood, poor sleep, decreased energy, decreased interest in sex, and changes in appetite all improve. However, these medications are not very useful for the treatment of pain.

The sedating tricyclic antidepressants such as amitriptyline, nortriptyline, or doxepin may prove useful to treat a sleep disturbance when no other symptoms of depression are present. These drugs are also much more useful for pain than the SSRIs.

Trazodone (Desyrel) is also useful for sleep disturbance, but it is not a good drug for pain, and is a mediocre drug for depression.

Antianxiety Medications

The most important forms of treatment for anxiety in patients with chronic neck pain are psychotherapy, relaxation training, biofeedback, and cognitive-behavioral training. Antianxiety medications can be helpful for short-term relief of anxiety, but are generally not good medications for long-term use.

However, antianxiety medications can be used to help sleep if the antidepressants have not worked. Clonazepam (Klonopin) can be useful in treating pain due to nerve damage and to treat some of the side effects of opioid analgesics.

18
Conclusions and Future Directions

A generation ago, most health care consumers placed all their faith in and expected absolute answers from their doctors, but things have changed. Most people now realize that doctors do not and cannot know everything, and no doctor is right all of the time. For those reasons, it is important for each person to take an active role in his or her own health care. Throughout this book, I've tried to emphasize that medicine is a constantly evolving art and science, with a constant stream of new information about most medical conditions, including neck pain. In the future, the way we evaluate and treat neck pain will combine the best research from biology, chemistry, and psychology, with the help of engineering, design, and principles of ergonomics. The emphasis will shift from the treatment of neck pain to prevention. Workplace design will be geared toward keeping workers healthy and more productive, not avoiding lawsuits.

Modern workers and homemakers will need to learn how to "work smart," especially when they are using computers and other high-tech equipment. In addition to learning how to work computers, we will be taught how to work in front of them. We will be taught how to set up our workstations at the office or at home, how to choose a good chair and desk, and how to use our furniture and equipment in ways that make ergonomic sense.

Changes in our health care system mean that patients will need to assume even more responsibility for their own care. In this era of managed health care and restrictive health insurance, doctors are inundated with paperwork to justify their diagnostic testing and treatment recommendations to insurance companies who are trying to minimize their expenditures. At the same time, doctors' reimbursements for the same amount of work are declining, and, as a result, doctors have less time to spend with each patient. So you must be prepared when you visit your doctors to be able to utilize your limited time well. To get the most from a visit, you can read books or magazine articles or search the Internet for educational materials about your condition. Keeping a written log of symptoms and a list of questions and concerns will allow you to get the most from your office visit. You can no longer rely completely on your doctor.

PREVENTION OF NECK PAIN

Neck pain affects a very large proportion of the population, and is getting more common. Among other things, neck pain can be caused by traumatic injuries and motor vehicle accidents. In our modern computer era, however, the most common cause of neck pain may be the cumulative trauma resulting from sitting at a desk with incorrect posture while working at a computer.

Despite its prevalence, neck pain need not be an inevitable part of the computer generation, and the scores of young people who spend hours playing or working at computers are not doomed to be in pain. Since neck pain is due to poor posture and body mechanics, not the computer per se, it is preventable. The concepts of treatment outlined in this book work very well as preventive measures. The problem is how to get people to take prevention seriously.

Pain is a great motivator. When you hurt, you will take the necessary measures and make the changes required to feel better. You will go to the gym and exercise, change your posture, and change your body mechanics at work and at play. But if you are not in pain, there is far less motivation to change bad habits. Furthermore, many of us live in a state of denial. We feel that we will always be healthy. It may never occur to us that the same illnesses and accidents that happen to others could happen to us. We sometimes rely more on luck than logic, and so it is hard to "sell" prevention.

Prevention is an interesting concept, because when it is successful, you can never really be sure that it worked. For example, consider the Y2K phenomenon. For at least eighteen months before the end of 1999, we heard a great deal about the terrible computer problems that might occur on January 1, 2000. We were bombarded with concerns about everything from air flight control to electricity and water supplies. We were warned about our bank accounts and the stock market. We were told to have emergency food, water, backup power sources, and cash on hand. But nothing happened.

In the days after the year 2000 began, some people were critical of government and industry, charging that the Y2K problem was overblown. But this is not true. We discovered the problem early, recognized what might occur, and took the necessary preventive measures. We checked out our computers, fixed the software problems, and then tested the corrections to be sure they worked. We practiced prevention. The problem was not overblown—prevention worked. The same could be said of neck pain. If you discover through reading this book, for example, that you use bad postures while typing, you might take steps to correct your posture. If you do not develop neck pain, was your concern unnecessary or were your preventive measures successful?

There are essentially two types of prevention in medicine. Primary prevention refers to the avoidance of a problem before it begins. Secondary prevention is the avoidance of future episodes once an initial episode of illness has occurred. Most of this book has dealt with secondary prevention—what to do after you've recovered from an initial episode of neck pain to prevent further episodes.

Paradoxically, the best hope for the future treatment of neck pain is primary prevention, not advances in diagnosis and treatment. We now know many of the factors that predispose a person for developing neck pain: poor posture, poor body mechanics, weak neck and back muscles, automobile head restraints that are too low, and more. Most of these contributing factors are under our control and can be corrected.

Chances are that if you are reading this book, you or someone you know has already been experiencing problems. But what about people who do not have neck pain, especially the next generation? We can begin to teach children in grade school and high school the basics of good posture for sitting, writing, reading, and working at computers. We can use gym class to teach exercises in ways that are fun. We can include instruction in posture and body mechanics in computer education courses. We can insist that new employees at computer-based jobs attend classes on body mechanics, and give them chairs and desks that fit well. The costs for education may be moderate in the short-term, but the future savings realized by avoiding health care costs, lost workdays, and disability payments will be well worth it. The savings in pain and suffering, of course, would be immeasurable.

Ergonomics of the "New" Workplace

The workplace is currently evolving. Although there are still many people who do traditional work, more and more of us have jobs that rely heavily on computers. As a result, we spend much more time sitting at desks, reading, entering data, keyboarding, and using a mouse. This has led to a marked increase in the incidence of neck pain. In order to reverse this trend, changes in the workplace, especially in the design of our chairs and desks, are necessary.

Desk chair design has been improving. Office chairs that adjust to various heights and angles are now available in every furniture store. There are chairs with built-in lumbar supports and chairs with high backs that offer neck support. However, instruction on how to use these chairs is not built in. Simply purchasing an ergonomic chair will not automatically ensure proper posture. Many people have expensive and well-designed chairs, but they use them so badly, they might as well be sitting on barstools. Take a look around a typical office setting. People tend to slump in their chairs, leaning forward over their work. They sit with poor posture—little or no lumbar curve, a hunched upper back, and neck sticking out and leaning down. Poor posture and body mechanics can render even an ergonomic chair ordinary. As outlined in chapter 9, concerning posture and body mechanics, using a chair well entails leaning against the back, sitting up straight, and working with good posture.

Unlike the innovations in chair design, there have been very few advances in the designs of desks and tables. Desks are usually available in only one height, and for many people, a desk of standard height does not fit well. Desks or tables with legs of adjustable lengths and whose tops can be adjusted to different angles to provide a more ergonomic surface for reading and writing would be two significant improvements. In fact, you can make these improvements yourself if your office is in your home.

Some people complain that ergonomic design does not look fashionable. Although you may have to make small sacrifices in aesthetics, your reward for using good ergonomic design will be better posture and better function. Soon, because form follows function, aesthetics will improve.

IMPROVED PROFESSIONAL EDUCATION

As you've learned in previous chapters, patients and consumers are not the only ones with things to learn about neck pain. Because of the explosion in medical research and information, health care professionals face an even more daunting challenge trying to keep up-to-date.

Physicians

Medicine changes very rapidly. It is difficult for physicians to keep current in their own specialty fields of interest, let alone subspecialties. Doctors rely more and more on journals that summarize information published elsewhere, especially for new information in fields outside their areas of expertise. Many spend their valuable continuing education time concentrating on diseases that are serious and life-threatening, and to them more interesting, than on common and seemingly mundane problems like neck pain or low back pain. Yet, neck and low back pain are two of the most common reasons people consult their primary care doctors. In fact, low back pain is second only to the common cold as a reason for visits to doctors, and neck pain is not far behind.

Given the prevalence of neck and back pain, it makes sense for medical review courses and textbooks to present better and more current information about these subjects. Doctors schooled in older theories do not have much to offer their patients with neck pain. But if they were shown that there were things they could do to help their patients, the subject would seem more interesting and exciting to them.

Another deficit in the professional education is that doctors are not usually well trained in the use of pain medications. Many doctors cling to old beliefs that analgesics are harmful, and should not be used for chronic pain. They are not trained to use antidepressants or other types of specialized analgesics effectively, despite the fact that pain is so widespread in our society. Continuing education should provide updates in these important areas.

Chiropractors

Chiropractors face a different problem, because if they are trained in a particularly rigid philosophy, it is very difficult for them to accept alternative theories of treatment. Some shun true science and remain dependent upon anecdotes. However, most chiropractic colleges are now teaching the scientific method, and many are including rehabilitation methods in addition to spinal manipulative therapy (SMT) in their curricula.

To ensure the greatest benefit to patients, chiropractors and medical doctors should work together and learn together, sharing ideas and opinions. Mutual education about their respective disciplines could occur if medical doctors lectured at chiropractic colleges and continuing education seminars, and chiropractors taught at medical schools and medical continuing education courses.

Physical Therapists

Many of the same gaps in the education of medical doctors and chiropractors are also present in the training and continuing education of physical therapists (PTs). The modern PT is a rehabilitation specialist who teaches exercise and body mechanics training, administers spinal manipulative therapy, and does workplace and injured worker evaluations. However, some therapists cling to older ideas and do only massage therapy, ice and heat treatments, and electrical muscle stimulation. These therapists would benefit from education in the current concepts of disorders of the spine, and some medical doctors would benefit from knowing how their PT colleagues have expanded their areas of expertise.

IMPROVED MEDICATIONS

At this time, there are no perfect medications to treat pain. Every medication choice requires balancing the potential for benefit against the risk of side effects. The most commonly used drugs, acetaminophen and the NSAIDs, are effective for mild to moderate pain. But they are somewhat unpredictable, in that they help some people but not others, even when they have what seems to be the same condition. They also have the potential for many side effects. The opioids are useful for acute pain, and may provide relief in some patients with severe, refractory (resistant to treatment) neck pain. However, they cause dependence and have many side effects. The muscle relaxants do not specifically relax muscles. They are more like sedatives, and can cause dependence. The antidepressants are very effective for depression, and may help some patients with chronic pain, but the results are not predictable. They also have the potential for many side effects.

However, the outlook for better pain medications is improving. There are many people with chronic pain who would derive benefit from better drugs. The pharmaceutical industry knows this and so is constantly searching for drugs that effectively relieve pain, have few or no side effects, and do not produce dependence. There is also a great deal of work being done to find better antidepressants. On the horizon are drugs that will specifically single out the receptors in the brain that can relieve pain and treat depression.

INTERNET SITES

An increasing number of physicians are interested in disorders of the spine, which has led to more good research about diagnosis and treatment. At each annual meeting of the North American Spine Society (NASS), there are over two hundred original research presentations. It is difficult for doctors to keep up with all this new information, and even more difficult for the public to be made aware of what is new and available to them.

As a clinician first and a researcher, teacher, and writer second, I try to keep up-to-date by reading medical journals, attending NASS meetings, and conferring with other physicians and researchers on a regular basis. I am also involved with two Web sites, the well-established *www.spinecare.com* and *www.neckpainbook.com*. I plan to post regularly any information about new advances in the field of neck pain on this Web site. I will post summaries of new research (called abstracts), and comment on them as well. In this way, readers can stay as up-to-date as their doctors. Some other reputable Web sites have been listed throughout this book and in appendix B.

NECK SURGERY

Artificial Discs

For many people, the disc is the weak link in the spinal motion chain. Under normal conditions, discs tend to wear out over the course of many years, but when they wear prematurely or are injured, there may be pain. The usual surgery for a degenerated disc has been removal of the disc and, when necessary, fusing together the vertebrae above and below. This, of course, makes the segment immobile and alters the mechanics of the neck. It would be desirable to keep motion normal, and one theoretical way to do this would be to replace a worn disc with an artificial disc.

Spine surgeons have worked to develop an artificial disc for many years. Many models have been tested in the laboratory, but only a few have ever worked well enough to even be tested in humans. To date, the only artificial disc implants have been in the lumbar spine. In Europe, there have been several thousand artificial discs implanted, but it is not yet possible to know if they work. The patients have not been observed for a long-enough time period and the surgeons have not been required to report their results for independent reviews. However, eventually, the artificial disc will be perfected for the low back, and then for the cervical spine.

Disc Transplants

Even more appealing than an artificial disc is a disc transplant. To date, there have been experiments in pigs in which a disc has been transplanted successfully from one part of its spine to another part, and was not rejected in the new disc space. Experiments with pig-to-pig disc transplants are under way. Up to now, there have not been experiments in humans. Perhaps eventually it will be possible to obtain discs, like corneas, from victims of trauma, and transplant them to others.

CONCLUSION

These are just a few of the directions that I foresee in the future for the field of neck pain, whiplash, and neck-related headache. I can assure the reader that there are very good scientists and medical doctors working to improve the care of our patients with neck pain.

Writing this book has been one of the most enjoyable and challenging things I have ever done. It has given me an opportunity to do the thing I like to do best—learn while teaching. I learned because I needed to be sure of everything I wrote. I looked up new references, reread old ones, and thought about many of the patients I had seen. I tried to remember some patients who got well and worried anew about some who didn't. I reflected on my work, and thought once again how I might do it better. Finally, I tried to write the way I try to talk to patients—clearly, and accurately, and in a way that is easily understood. I hope I was successful.

Appendix A
Selected Readings

Angell, M., and J. P. Kassirer. "Alternative Medicine. The Risks of Untested and Unregulated Remedies." *Skeptical Inquirer* 23(1999):58–60.

Two editors of the prestigious *New England Journal of Medicine* feel that what sets alternative medicine apart from conventional medicine is that it has not been scientifically tested for safety or efficacy. Its advocates deny the need for such testing, and instead practitioners rely on anecdotes and theories.

Beyerstein, B. L. "Why Bogus Therapies Seem to Work." *Skeptical Inquirer* (September/October 1997).

This article explores the many reasons that therapies that are not really effective appear to help. It is very thought-provoking.

Cassileth, B. R. *The Alternative Medicine Handbook: The Complete Reference Guide to Alternative and Complementary Therapies.* New York: W. W. Norton & Co., 1998.

The book gives a very balanced look at a range of complementary and alternative therapies, and reviews what the claims are for each, as well as any existing scientific studies. The major subjects are spiritual healing, dietary and herbal remedies, manual therapy, and others.

Catalano, E. M., and K. N. Hardin. *The Chronic Pain Control Workbook.* Oakland: New Harbinger Publications, 1996.

This is an excellent book on pain written by people who are very experienced in the field. There are many "self-help" suggestions that are worth considering.

Cranz, G. *The Chair: Rethinking Culture, Body, and Design.* New York: W. W. Norton & Co., 1998.

This book by an architect reviews the cultural, aesthetic, and ergonomics of chairs. It is a fun book to read with many interesting insights about how form may not always follow function.

Homola, S., and S. Barrett. *Inside Chiropractic: A Patient's Guide.* Amherst, NY: Prometheus Books, 1999.

This book, written by a chiropractor, exposes the negative side of chiropractic, but also discusses how to find a good chiropractor who can help neck and low back pain.

Linden, P. *Compute in Comfort.* Upper Saddle River, NJ: Prentice Hall, 1995.

One of many good books on working at a computer. Quite readable and comprehensive.

McKenzie, R. *Treat Your Own Neck.* Waikanae, New Zealand: Spinal Publications, 1983.

Robin McKenzie has made great contributions to the treatment of low back and neck pain. His book describes the exercises for acute neck pain, but it does not discuss the details of the causes of pain.

Melton, M. *The Guide to Whiplash.* Olympia, WA: Body-Mind Publications, 1998.

This is a review of the symptoms and signs of whiplash injury written for the public. It is very well researched and referenced.

Sinel, M. S., W. W. Deardorff, and T. B. Goldstein. *Win the Battle Against Back Pain.* New York: Dell Books, 1996.

This is a comprehensive book on low back pain. Many of the insights and suggestions apply equally well to neck pain.

Appendix B
Health Care Resources

Medical Practices

SpineCare Medical Group
San Francisco Spine Institute, 1850 Sullivan Avenue, #200, Daly City, CA 94015, (650) 985-7500, *www.spinecare.com*.
   A comprehensive spine center for the diagnosis and treatment of neck and low back pain. Multidisciplinary team of doctors who specialize in operative and nonoperative care. Includes surgeons, injection specialists, pain management specialists, and psychiatrists.

Web Sites

The Cervicogenic Headache Institute, *www.headpain.com*.
   A private practice of primarily surgeons who treat many patients with neck-related headaches.
SpineCare Medical Group, *www.spinecare.com*.
   A user-friendly format that answers most of the pertinent questions of people with spinal pain.
The World Cervicogenic Headache Society, *www.cervicogenic.com*.
   A Web site with information about neck-related headaches.

Organizations

American Chronic Pain Association
P.O. Box 850, Rocklin, CA 95677, (916) 632-0922, *www.theacpa.org*.

An excellent self-help organization that provides much-needed information about dealing with chronic pain.

Back to Golf, *www.backtogolf.com.*
A physical therapy network whose members are specially trained to treat golfers with back or neck pain.

North American Spine Society
22 Calendar Court. #200, LaGrange, IL 60525, *www.spine.org.*
The leading organization of doctors and other health professionals dedicated to the diagnosis and treatment of the spine.

Products to Help Your Neck: Chairs, Pillows, Headsets, etc.

Aqua-Jogger belt (available in many sports equipment stores)
A belt that allows you to float vertically in the water, and thereby exercise effectively.

BackSaver Products
53 Jeffrey Avenue, Holliston, MA 01746–9865, (800) 251-2225.
A catalog business that sells high-quality ergonomic chairs, chair side tables, foam wedges, and much more. They are part of Relax the Back Stores.

Hello Direct
5893 Rue Ferrari, San Jose, CA 95138–1857, (800) 444-3556, *www.hellodirect.com.*
A maker of good-quality headsets and telephone-related equipment.

Pain Reliever.com, *www.painreliever.com.*
An on-line vendor for many products that are helpful for neck pain. They have many types of pillows and other products.

Plantronics
8320 Hedge Lane Terrace, Shawnee, KS 62227, (800) 882-7779, *www.plantronics.com.*
    A maker of high-quality headsets, especially the Plantronics PLX 400 headset and phone supplies.

Alternative and Complementary Medicine

American Association of Acupuncture and Oriental Medicine, (610) 266-1433.

American Massage Therapy Association
820 Davis Street, Suite 100, Evanston, IL 60201, (847) 864-0123, *www.amtamassage.org.*

National Center for Complementary and Alternative Medicine, *www.nccam.nih.gov.*

Index